HEALTH IN THE NEW AGE

HEALTH IN THE NEW AGE

A STUDY IN CALIFORNIA HOLISTIC PRACTICES

J. A. English-Lueck

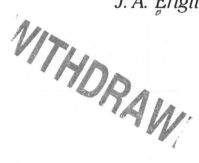

University of New Mexico Press

ALBUQUERQUE

To June English (1920–1987),

who taught me to respect

history and delight in people

Library of Congress Cataloging-in-Publication Data

English-Lueck, J. A. (June Anee), 1953–
    Health in the new age : a study of California holistic
practices / J. A. English-Lueck. — 1st ed.
      p.   cm.
    Includes bibliographical references.
    ISBN 0–8263–1177–6
    1. Holistic medicine—California 2. New Age move-
ment—California. I. Title.
    R733.E54 1990
    613'.09794—dc20   89–38848
                                     CIP

Design by Susan Gutnik.

C O N T E N T S

ACKNOWLEDGMENTS

It is almost impossible to thank everyone who helped me produce this book and maintain my balance for the duration. My husband, Karl Lueck, deserves the lion's share of such thanks. He patiently advised and assisted me during my fieldwork. He read and edited all my drafts. Most of all, he gave me emotional and financial support when I needed it. He and my mother, June English, took care of my beloved toddler Miriam while I spent many long hours editing. Special thanks go to the English and Lueck clans for their understanding.

I acknowledge my debts for the academic support and criticisms of Paul Bohannan, William Madsen, John Platt, and Barbara Voorhies. In addition, I would like to thank Robert Textor, Ruth Moore, and Dirk van der Elst for their additional intellectual stimulation.

I wish to thank the understanding and supportive employers who allowed me to work undisturbed by financial anxieties. This includes: the Anthropology department at the University of California, Santa Barbara; Pandora Snethkamp and the Office of Public Archaeology, Santa Barbara; P-III Associates; the department of Comparative Sociology, University of Puget Sound; and the department of Anthropology at California State University, Fresno, and the Intensive Language Centre at the Chengdu University of Science and Technology in the People's Republic of China.

I wish to express my appreciation for the large personal support network that kept me enthusiastic and inspired in this task. These peers, colleagues, and friends gave me ideas and emotional support that went beyond my expectations. A brief list includes Barbara Leavitt, Veeda Marchetti, Linda Beth Freese, Joanne Kipps, Denise Roberts, Enos Njeru, Tom Conelly, Miriam Chaiken, Jim and Terry Rudolph, Craig and Lorraine Woodman, Randall Luce, Jerry Moore, Greg and Eilene Cross, Geri Morales, George Guilmet, and the secretarial staff at UCSB.

I would especially like to thank the editorial staff at the University of New Mexico Press for their patience and their help. Their careful guidance has enhanced the book immeasurably. Finally, I wish to thank the holistic health community. Although I cannot thank them by name, I appreciate their cooperation, honesty, and insight. They brought a special joy to the work.

INTRODUCTION

Between the Mountains and the Sea,

Paraiso[1] *is a Place for Healing.*

(Selinsky 1982: 1)

HOLISTIC HEALERS: AN ETHNOGRAPHY

California has been a Mecca for a variety of social and technical revolutions, including the "Aquarian conspiracy." First coined by Marilyn Ferguson, the Aquarian conspiracy referred to a conscious attempt to reform Western society, centered around the symbol of the new age of Aquarius (Ferguson 1980: 19). The new age movement included many diverse goals. Members of the social movement deliberately sought to promote values of self-responsibility, plural lifestyles, psychological growth, creativity, affection, and a sense of ecological connection (Bloomfield 1978: 272–3; Mattson 1982: 41). The holistic health experience was a key catalyst in recruiting for the Aquarian movement (Ferguson 1980: 257).

Holistic health has seldom been the primary focus of published anthropological work. Major exceptions to this include the work of Mattson on Bay Area holistic health practitioners (1977; 1982), and Grossinger's analysis of healing, especially homeopathy (1980). In addition, several dissertations have addressed similar subjects. Molgaard worked with a New Age community in the Northwest (1979) and Galanti produced an informative analysis of psychics in Los Angeles (1981). The approach of this book independently parallels Mattson's in many ways, focusing on questions of the future of holistic health as a movement. I hope we augment and complement each other.

---

[1] Community and individual practitioner names have been changed to insure confidentiality.

In the past, the holistic health movement has been poorly understood outside of the networks of its own community. As an anthropologist immersing myself in the beliefs, practices, and values of the holistic health community, I can provide a unique point of view, describing the movement from the insider's and outsider's perspective. My major task is to explain the continuity of an alternative tradition in a complex society. In seeking an explanation of how a minority tradition survives and sometimes flourishes, three themes emerged. First, even in a seemingly novel movement, there is a long legacy of historical tradition. Second, as historical factors change, new concepts and practices restructure the legacy, and new ideas become part of the tradition. Third, flexible social structures allow the tradition to persist and yet permit change. Decentralized, egalitarian groups maintain the tradition and are hard to eliminate. When circumstances permit, the movement becomes more formally organized. In holistic health, the tradition is derived from thousands of years of naturalistic medicine—medical systems based primarily on the balance of metaphysical forces (elements and life forces). Historical factors have reshaped the ideas that are now present in holistic health. The continuity is maintained by the dispersed, decentralized nature of the practitioners. Small groups of individuals can persist where large organizations might not survive. At the same time, however, the 1980s may see the growth of professionalism in the movement.

Holistic health represents a clear example of a social movement, linked, allied, or opposed to the rest of the community in a complex fashion. This changing community is part of a larger social movement, introducing countercultural values and rejecting the dominant views of orthodox medicine and traditional authority. The holistic health movement is not simply a group of people favoring one health care system over the prevailing paradigm, however, but an ideological community actively pursuing a desired future. My major task was to draw out the hoped for realities from the practitioners. The created ideology not only formed a pattern for behavior, it did so by consciously seeking a particular future.

My goal has been to produce an ethnography of the community of people who define themselves as holistic health practitioners. The ethnographic field tradition in anthropology is a broadly based, analytic translation of the daily experience of human beings living in a specific setting. Each segment of activity is described; the segments are linked together in a way that makes the reader understand how the parts interact. An ethnography should also allow an informant to understand his/her world as an outsider might see it, and still communicate to an outsider the "inside view" of that culture. Such translation uses the scientific models of the time as decoders.

No finer model of ethnographic style can be found than the classic work *Coral Gardens and Their Magic* by Bronislaw Malinowski (1978, originally 1935). It presents all the elements of ethnography. The focus is direct and concrete. It examines gardens in the Trobriand Islands of Melanesia, drawing connections with economic specialization, fishing, settlement patterns, land tenure, kinship, political structure, exchange systems, garden magic, and linguistics. In drawing these connections to "describe" the Coral Gardens, Malinowski was creating anthropological theory. If the basic assumption of anthropology is true, and culture is integrated and interconnected, we can approach the whole of that society through one aspect. Even the most comprehensive description can thus be problem oriented. The description must branch out from its focal point and examine related phenomena.

Modern ethnographies can still use this method of integrating information. Malinowski's specific categories are not appropriate for all projects, and certainly not for holistic healers in California in the eighties. Yet his style—painting a large picture through the interpretation of a specific detail is the essence of ethnography.

There was a time when anthropologists found it difficult to recognize the complexity of "Primitives." As they learned more, they discovered enormous individual variation (Bohannan 1963: 22). In spite of these variations, it is possible to study a peasant village. Complex societies offer their own challenges of diversity and amazing intricacy, but it should be possible to construct an ethnography of aspects of modern America, focusing at one point and noting the variety.

Since the time of Malinowski, ethnographic tradition has remained coherent through many changes. Current fieldwork techniques are remarkably similar to those used by Malinowski. Even as it has been enhanced by decades of experience, the core of cultural anthropological fieldwork remains participant observation, living with a people while observing their behavior. Anthropology still uses concepts borrowed from biology and psychology to develop interpretive schema. The anthropological models, our cultural decoders, have changed in detail, not in kind.

An ethnography of holistic healers requires a focus that incorpo-
rates the interpretive models that reflect the state of anthropology in
the 1980s: the interaction of the individual and society through time,
from the past, through the ethnographic present, and projected into the
future. The focus of this study is the idea of the social movement. This
is the mechanism by which individuals change their society and are
changed by the new concepts it provides. It cannot be clearly perceived synchronically, for it is a phenomenon of change over time.

A medical system is a fit subject for the study of values and assumptions because it closely reflects the basic assumptions and attitudes of the parent society. If the cultural cosmology is populated by
spirits of varying malevolence, the medical belief system reflects it. If
the universe is seen as a dynamic flux of forces, elements, energies,
and humors, the medical system reflects this world view (Foster and
Anderson 1978: 51–79, Treacher and Wright 1982: 11–12). If the cosmology consists of separable causes and effects, then it should come
as no surprise when the medical system reflects this rationalist paradigm. The logic of holistic health reflects the values and beliefs that
are part of the larger New Age movement.

In order to reveal the values & beliefs of the holistic community I
had to develop techniques that penetrated routine behavior and elic-
ited values. These values should echo the perceptions of what holistic
healers think is going on in the world and what can and should be
done about it. This involves the intricate operation of separating an
ethnographer's values from those of the holistic health community. Although others were also used; the most important technique of this
study was participant observation.

Fieldwork is a rite of passage often described in anthropological
literature—*Return to Laughter* (Bowen 1964), *Diary in the Strict Sense
of the Term* (Malinowski 1967), *Letters from the Field 1925–1975* (Mead
1977), and others in this genre (Agar 1980; Powdermaker 1967; Wax
1971). My own experience began with brief but meaningful fieldwork in
Surinam among the Kwinti Maroons and in Holland. However, the problems of working as an anthropologist in my own culture are distinct.

When the degree of divergence between home culture and study
culture is great, observation comes almost of itself. Studying a familiar
culture requires another kind of vigilance and constant analytical awareness (Albon 1977). Just as it would be difficult for me to honestly evalu-

ate and analyze my family and peers, I found it hard to isolate my feelings for the holistic health community. The holistic health community included people I cared about and respected, and yet I had to acknowledge the presence in their world view of particular contradictions, social traps, and historical inconsistencies that make up any human behavior. I had to school myself to recognize historical processes at work beyond my attitudes.

Thus, my initial assumptions proved to be naive. I had assumed that growing up in California was sufficient preparation for me to work with the holistic health community with a minimum of introductory fieldwork. Moreover, I felt I could separate my life into convenient compartments and so maintain my "objectivity." The barriers of my own assumptions had to be crossed to complete my fieldwork.

My personal and academic life bore the brunt of breakdowns in my attempts at compartmentalization. Early in the fieldwork a practitioner I was working with explained that celibacy was a strict rule for the period of instruction and therapy—about two months. My husband felt that was taking participant observation too far! Yet how could I stop my enculturation into the holistic community at my front door? Luckily, my husband is a tolerant fellow, and I discovered I could not always follow instructions. Such conflicts became even more acute in the professional sphere, particularly when my schedule demanded that I submerge myself in the holistic community during the mornings and evenings and redirect my attention to teaching rationalist academic anthropology in the afternoons. The crisis came eighteen months into the fieldwork. I was working a few hours a week as an ombudsman in a university clinic, mediating conflicts between the very orthodox staff and the student patients. When the students demanded more holistic medicine, to the horror of the staff, my compartmentalization self-destructed. The conflict too closely mirrored my own internal battle. I had to withdraw from the position, unable to betray the holistic world-view while I was still immersed in my fieldwork.

Conflict was not, however, the dominant theme in my personal relations with the community. I was genuinely intrigued and often helped by their teachings. Halfway through my fieldwork my father contracted terminal cancer. My mother-in-law and father died within a month of each other. My network of practitioners rallied to my aid, giving me the techniques to explore and cope with my grief, allowing me to find some balance during a difficult time. The community always seemed to know I was an incorrigible rationalist but accepted and educated me anyway.

I was taught that there are many small differences in meaning and behavior that are essential in understanding the rich diversity of the holistic health community. Word meanings, physical space, literary and personal references, and values are all subtly distinct from those outside the holistic health community. For example, in the holistic health sphere "energy" is a phenomenon that is subjectively experienced. A holistic health practitioner intuitively "feels energy." That concept is distinctly different from the objective, easily quantified power source of the outside society. Understanding the medical belief system, as well as the set of rules governing acceptable interpersonal behavior took some time. Even straightforward tasks such as census taking were elusively complex. Individual practitioners are highly mobile and often necessarily maintain a low profile. In short, I learned to appreciate that the holistic health community is as rich and diverse as any foreign village and I needed to redefine my expectations.

A major difficulty existed in conveying the information I had obtained. In order to protect the privacy of my informants, I was reluctant to divulge many of the details that are found in traditional ethnographies. To solve this dilemma, I concentrated on the beliefs and practices of the practitioners. Personal details are used sparingly, only if needed to illustrate attitudes or social dynamics.

The observations that underlie this study come from two years' fieldwork in the holistic health networks of a city in Southern California. I took one year to survey the groups and individuals practicing one or more of the techniques considered by the practitioners to be the domain of holistic health. I sought out workshops, classes, institutes, professional and avocational meetings, private therapists, and health oriented living collectives. I then spent nine months attending an eclectic training institute for holistic health practitioners, which provided invaluable information for understanding the relationship between a social movement and the individual. Within this facility, novice healers not only learned a wealth of techniques, but the philosophies that linked the practices together. In addition, students were introduced to concepts of "professionalism" and were exposed to legal and political organizations and networks.

In this setting, values and expected behavior were carefully and clearly articulated. There were frequent discussions and speculations on the goals of the Aquarian movement and the personal and global futures that will create it. At the same time I began to gather a small sample of interviews including standardized questions about education, upbringing, medical histories, life-styles, and goals. This was followed by biographical sketches based on the life events important in becoming a holistic health practitioner.

Another method that was helpful in revealing underlying assumptions and goals was the Ethnographic Futures Research technique (EFR). Eliciting cultural premises is the primary goal of EFR and I found it useful in two ways. Initially, I used EFR purely as an interview technique. Coupled with my biographic sketches, I encouraged the practitioners to describe scenarios of the best, worst, and most probable futures in the next twenty-five to thirty years, within the bounds of what they think is possible. I encouraged them to tell me the factors on which these futures hinged (Textor 1980: 38, 44). I was most interested in getting the practitioners' ideas about the future, as well as overall state of the world.

The concepts in EFR also proved useful in organizing my observational notes, as well as vocational handbooks, commonly used inspirational Aquarian novels, and public documents such as contracts, newsletters, advertisements, and statements of purpose. Submerged in each of these messages are ambiguous warnings against the worst future, visions of the best, and ideas of the most probable scenario. Using EFR categories made such classifications more explicit.

The areas of future practice and global transformation were categories that occurred naturally in the interview process. They were issues consciously developed in the minds of holistic health practitioners. Healers felt a sense of urgency. They believed that current choices concerning profession and life-style would transform their lives within the next twenty-five years.

Practitioners' future scenarios break down into concerns of health care and the state of the world. The latter are characterized by different conscious goals. These aims may be nativistic, harkening back to a Golden Age; they may be revitalizing syntheses or millenial global transformations in which the old order would be destroyed and a new order, a New Age would ensue. There are indications that modern social movements contain all these ideas. Such movements are social networks linked by media-borne ideology. Visions of the future provide a focus for group leadership and group cohesion. The thematic unity of the holistic health practitioners' views of the future reveals important social processes. The diversity among the practitioners points to issues that form the basis of the fissioning of the community into smaller groups.

Using EFR, practitioners are asked to present "realistic" scenarios. The guideline of "realism" is itself provocative. It reveals the concepts that individuals form as to what constitutes legitimate process. Individuals believe that their personal professional choices will realistically determine whether or not the holistic health movement is absorbed by cosmopolitan, allopathic medicine. Processes such as "karma" or "global spiritual evolution" are perceived as natural rather than extravagant agents of change. "Realism" hints at the assumptions permitting visions of medical plurality and millennial transformation.

Beyond the content, even the structure of the scenarios can be analysed. Some holistic health practitioners envision three distinct scenarios. Best, worst, and most probable futures are not overlapping. Each has a separate reality. Yet this is not the only way to perceive the future. There can also be a unified vision of the future, in which the best and worst scenarios are the most probable, and all would happen. My own bias was in seeing scenarios as "best" or "worst", or some synthesis of each. It had not occurred to me that some individuals would be so secure in their anticipation of the future, or commitment to that future, that they would have one unified scenario.

I noticed this rare conception occurred only among the major leaders of the community. This particular vision may be very useful in creating charismatic rapport with holistic health novices and practitioners. The disasters of the worst case usher in the new age of the best scenario. Linking disaster and terrestrial spiritual transformation and developing unified cognitive maps of the future are two features of millennialism which I would not have seen without the EFR technique.

THE ETHNOGRAPHIC FOCUS:
THE SEQUENCE OF
A SOCIAL MOVEMENT

There are two major tasks in developing the problem underlying this study. The first is descriptive—defining the nature of the holistic health community, delineating the range of practices, and outlining networks. Current and historical assumptions, organization, and practices of individual practitioners are important in understanding both common features and diversity. Chapters 2, 3, and 4 address this line of inquiry. This descriptive effort provides the background for development of a theoretical framework that helps organize the wealth of ethnographic and historical observations of the holistic health movement. The analysis uses a model of social movements to explore how a social movement, lacking formal organization, survives in society. This analysis is the second major task. Chapters 5, 6, and 7 are devoted to that mission.

Chapters 2 and 3 explore the contemporary expression of holistic health, outlining social organization as well as the diverse range of beliefs and practices. This diversity demands some explanation, however. What were the historical events that led to the creation of the beliefs and practices in holistic health? Such roots extend far beyond the rhetoric of the 1960s. Holistic health is a cross-cultural and historical synthesis, a descendent of powerful, ancient medical and philosophical traditions. Holistic health has reunited the common assumptions of the great naturalistic medical systems of the Old World—Asian, Ayurvedic, and Hippocratic traditions.

Issues arose historically that still have an impact on current holistic health concerns. Within the Hippocratic tradition, empiricism contains many of the assumptions that are today unique to holistic health and distinct from rationalist, cosmopolitan medicine. This philosophical position was reflected in the Christian esoteric tradition of Medieval and Renaissance Europe. Transcendentalism and Spiritualism added to the philosophical basis of holistic health, just as traditions of herbalism and self-help added to its practical basis in early America. Finally, holistic health is linked in alliance with and opposition to the influx of social movements that began in the 1930s and was reinforced in the 1960s. Understanding this complex of historical antecedents makes one see that the key concepts of holistic health are much more consistent with the Euro-American cultural tradition than it would appear at first glance.

Chapters 2, 3, and 4 provide the background necessary for discussing theoretical issues. From that edifice, in chapters 5, 6, and 7, I will branch out into the theoretical issues related to a social movement—

adaptation and social change; socialization and commitment; and the formation of professionalism, institutions, and the countercultural alternatives.

The generalized life cycle of a social movement (see Figure 1.1). relates to each of these issues. The model helps coordinate diverse issues into a single framework. A social movement might be born if a social problem is defined and partially solved by a key figure, often a charismatic leader who is referred to as a catalyst. If the analysis of the problem is borne out by events in reality and the analysis is communicated, members may be attracted to the movement. Often fissions occur, and constructive reanalyses are made that influence the direction of the movement, laying the foundation for the creation of an institution. Portions of the movement may also be driven "underground," as succeeding analyses diversify the movement.

The life cycle of a social movement is an organizing principle, and not an explanatory construct. The descriptive model does not reveal why a movement is necessary, where the initial statement of problem and solution came from, how individuals are attracted and initiated into a movement, or why some movements institutionalize and others retain an informal, grassroots social network. However, without a descriptive framework, any questions are difficult to ask.

As a social movement, holistic health plays with both new ideas and old ones in a new context. If culture is indeed the microadaptive mechanism of the human species, allowing us to change the way we live without complex genetic alterations, then new perceptions of behavioral alternatives and ideas are the analogues to biological variation—the basis of natural selection. Like genetic variation, these ideas must come from somewhere. In this context, any historical examination of a social movement is a close-range study of cultural variation and has the potential for evolutionary cultural changes of various orders of magnitude.

The organic, homeostatic model of culture popular in Malinowski's age was certainly useful, but biological models have become more sophisticated. Adding the dimension of time, evolutionary and ecological concepts can be cautiously borrowed from biology. New perspectives are created by introducing the concept of temporal change. At the same time, it is vital to remember that humans excel at creating and pursuing conscious goals. This is a fundamentally different phenomenon than biological adaptation. Examining human cultural change re-

FIGURE 1.1   THE SEQUENCE OF A SOCIAL MOVEMENT

1. *There must be a problem, a set of difficulties to be resolved.*
   - These can be social, ecological and personal, but must be perceived as having no solution in the status quo.

2. *A catalytic analysis is made. Someone makes a statement about the problem.*
   - There must be a historical basis—a background to present knowledge
   - There must be an "analyst"

3. *A crisis occurs, demonstrating the "truth" of the catalytic analysis.*
   - The crisis must be perceived as such and used to demonstrate the solution that is offered

4. *Members are gathered.*
   - Individuals must learn how to be members
   - Groups must unite in ideological networks
   - The ideology must provide a template for future action and reinforce the need to take action–

     Example: A millenarian movement is designed to transform the "real world" into utopia with the help of the supernatural. It depends on a perception of disaster joined with the hope of a new age. The Aquarian ideal is the basis of millenial hopes in the holistic health community.

5. *Constructive analyses are made.*
   - These form the basis for professional growth and the formation of new groups, institutionalised and informal.

6. *Policies are formed and institutions are developed.*
   - The holistic healers must quickly professionalize or be absorbed or destroyed in an economic conflict with "orthodox" medicine.

7. *Informal networks are maintained sub rosa.*

quires the examination of both the principles of adaptation and the range of consciously desired futures.

In many ways, the concept of the social movement is logically similar to a model of ecological adaptation. While they certainly make understanding phenomena much simpler, they are not adequate causal explanations. Both are models of "selection by consequences." The

behavior or form is shaped by the environment, influenced by feedback that occurs after the act. The kangaroo rat does not evolve water
conservative mechanisms because he lives in the desert. The rat's survival is shaped by the consequences of the environmental success of
his already existing form. If he is not water conservative, he will not
survive to reproduce. In both biological adaptation and social movements, there is "goal-seeking behavior," but that goal does not create
the behavior. It merely shapes it through later feedback. This is the nature of selection by consequences, whether in learning, natural selection, or social change (Skinner 1981). Bee wings were not created because the creature needed to fly, yet fins were clearly inappropriate!
Successful social movements do not arise each time a culture is no
longer adaptive, but lacking functional alternatives, the movements do
provide grist for the mill, a form to shape and adapt (see Salmon 1982:
89 and Salmon and Salmon 1979: 71). Evolution and social movements
do not cause changes, they are change (Rindos 1984: 39). Social movements cannot, per se, explain the acts of the individual members.

Naturally, human beings complicate this process further. Not only
do societies have complicated systems with ambiguous innate goals,
they consciously create new goals. People develop their own conscious aims and act to fulfill them. This means that humanity can act
on two separate levels of goal-seeking behavior. One is adaptive in an
evolutionary sense, the other is consciously Lamarckian (Rindos 1984:
73–79). Creating their own goals, individuals in a social movement
can define their own proximate causes (Salmon 1982: 88). Human beings can will change.

As a model of phenomena, a social movement may not in itself explain, but it provides questions and implications for consideration (Le
Blanc 1973: 207–212; Salmon 1982: 93). Using such a model as an explanation can be a trap. Such an explanation runs: "Social movements
occur because they are needed. Social movements create social change.
We know they do, because there is social change!" Logically, we know
this is misleading. It is not legitimate to use a consequence as a cause.
There can certainly be a need for social change without the appearance of a social movement. There can also be social movements that
accomplish nothing. All of these things led me to reject the concept
"social movement" as an explanation but to retain it as a useful descriptive model.

The interplay between form and purpose in a social movement are explored in chapter 5. The historical continuity outlined in chapter 4 has been molded by shifts in social design and purpose. In the holistic health movement these purposes unfold as different social goals, expressed in different social organizations. For example, "spiritual freedom" may be a goal that expresses itself as resistance to organized forms. Social organizations exist for a major ideological purpose and yet possess a number of more narrowly focused goals. These latter goals often determine if the movement will be classified as nativistic, revitalizing, or millenial. There is a difference between a "spiritual freedom" never previously experienced and one based on the wisdom of the ancient ones. They can all co-exist, however, within the framework of a larger ideological purpose. The discussion in chapter 5 on social movements is primarily based on the ideas of Margaret Mead (1964), John Platt (1975), A. F. C. Wallace (1956), Luther Gerlach (1980; Gerlach and Hine 1973; 1981) and Virginia Hine (1980)—ideas synthesized in the representation of the life cycle of a social movement.

In addition, well-documented historical movements are used to illustrate relevant issues. In particular, the early history of Christianity provides rich illustrations of the broad historical patterns in a social movement. Early Christianity demonstrates the diversity possible, even within a fully institutionalized social movement. In addition, not only did Christianity play a part in the antecedents of the holistic health movement itself, it documents the long periods of time involved in the cycles of a social movement. Few social movements have been analysed in such depth, or for such a long time, as Christianity.

The role of the individual is the dominant theme of chapter 6, exploring the processes of individual commitment and socialization. Perceptual unease, and the resolution of that dissonance by the ideals of a social movement, are matters of individual choice and learning. Learning in a personalistic and naturalistic medical system, as a profession/art, requires a special process, different from education in rationalistic medicine—less clinical and more like an apprenticeship. In addition to technical skills, the values of the movement are internalized during the training of a potential holistic health practitioner. These include the ability to make cognitive shifts in perception that channel empathy and intuition. The theoretical social, cognitive, and biological mechanisms of learning and methods of practice are explored in chapter 6.

Not every social movement becomes the basis of a new way of life, nor is every one lost in obscurity. What are the factors that lead to institutionalization or continued covert activity in a social movement? This is the focus of the seventh, and final chapter.

The professional direction of a practitioner is a matter of individual choice. The sum of those choices will be reflected in the fate of the movement. Professional choices vary, based on the degree of linkage to the medical establishment. If it becomes possible to establish a separate professional identity, a holistic health practitioner can exist autonomously. If the holistic health movement is co-opted by the medical establishment, there will only be the choices of becoming part of the medical establishment, remaining a covert esoteric tradition, or forming holistic medicine, in which the two positions are mixed. Politics, economic realities, and social traps are outside variables that influence individual decisions in this matter.

It is important to understand that holistic health is not an isolated phenomenon in this regard. Creation of health care alternatives is a process that is increasingly seen in the developed world. In medical anthropology, much effort has been spent in understanding the range of medical choice in the Third World, as cosmopolitan medicine enters and dominates the picture. Yet, there is a another side to this coin: in the developed world, revivals and syntheses of old traditions are springing up to fill the social gaps left by what is often perceived of as impersonal and expensive treatment. The choices made by individual holistic health practitioners, their allies, and opponents will shape medical plurality in America.

HOLISTIC HEALTH PRACTITIONERS

The bond that links your true family is not one of blood, but of respect and joy in each other's life. Rarely do members of one family grow up under the same roof. (*Illusions,* Bach 1984: 84)

Outside their own community, holistic health practitioners are not well understood. There are many misconceptions about them, derived from ideas about "quacks," "massage parlours," and "spacey Californians" that have little to do with their reality. To understand their lifestyle, let alone their community structure, it is necessary to convey a sense of their actual medical beliefs and practices. Initially, it is important to present some of the basic tenets of the holistic approach. A composite, hypothetical therapeutic interview, an actual client/practitioner session, illustrates the content of practices involved in holistic health. Along with the next chapter, this one provides the background for the description of the holistic health community as a social phenomenon.

OVERVIEW OF HOLISTIC HEALTH

Human potential is a fundamental concept in holistic health. In the Aquarian ideology, the healing and growth processes must extend beyond the individual body, but personal growth cannot go beyond the

limitations of the social environment. This means that for the individual to be truly well, society must be transformed. The holistic health
movement is made up of two interconnected aspects. Holistic health is
a symbol, containing moral codes—values referring to what life should
be. The valued states include freedom from pain, passion, and self-
ishness, and a state of serenity, honesty, and creativity. There is also a
commitment to "wellness," meaning spiritual attunement with natural
and social environments, as well as physical health (Mattson 1977: 36;
1982: 9). Responding to a question on the meaning of holistic health,
one holistic health practitioner pointed out that the root of *holistic* is
"kalos," a Greek root from which stems *health, whole,* and *holy.* He
said all were necessary for a true sense of well-being. The term symbolically links various practitioners who respond to "holistic health"
as a keyword trigger, signifying the introduction of spirituality into all
aspects of life.

Holistic health is also a set of techniques oriented to enacting
Aquarian ideals. Diagnostic tools include iridology, based on the appearance of the iris; aura analysis, sensing the psychic field around the
body; personology, a system of physical trait analysis; Asian based
pulse reading; and "Touch for Health." The latter uses muscle response
as it reflects acupuncture meridians. Therapies embrace Gestalt, Reichian, and Polarity therapies, applied kinesiology (Touch for Health and
Orthobionomy), homeopathy, chiropractic, naturopathy and herbology, movement and creative therapies, massage and bodywork, acupuncture, acupressure, and various nutritional regimens. An individual
practitioner in Paraiso may use one or all of these techniques. For example, a *shiatsu* masseuse may just use the techniques specific to that
discipline. Another person, trained at an eclectic academy, may use
iridology, applied kinesiology, and visual cues to guide therapy. Therapy might include dietary change, lifestyle counseling, and shiastu.
Both are still holistic health practitioners.

These techniques and others are syntheses of twentieth-century innovations based on three medical traditions that have survived millen-
nia: Asian, Ayurvedic, and Hippocratic/Unani. The Asian medical system focuses on energy flow, and the importance of food, feelings, and
social environment in establishing harmony. Similarly, the Indian Ayurvedic tradition contributed the idea of *chakras,* nodes of control that
regulate energy through endocrinological changes. Ayurvedic healing

emphasizes diet, yogic physical disciplines, and the maintenance of balance with the elements of the environment. Hippocratic concepts provide the basis for naturopathy (drugless techniques using diet, exercise, and massage to promote healing), homeopathy, and chiropractic. Recent innovations such as orthomolecular medicine promoted the use of megavitamin doses and are liberally mixed with the ancient traditions. Along with a smattering of Native American or Asian shamanic beliefs, these traditions form the backbone of holistic health practices. The practices are coupled with philosophies stemming from American Transcendentalism and natural mysticism; they focus on spiritual growth. The philosophies are usually brought to the movement by practitioners involved in humanistic and popular psychology, "New Thought" beliefs, such as Religious Science, and popular metaphysical/theosophical concepts.

Fusions of these approaches form a template for the diverse, individualised practices in holistic health. Communication of these highly personal beliefs and practices in a larger social sphere is the essence of the movement. The assumptions (see Figure 2.1) are vital in understanding the common values of movement members. There are, of course, many more assumptions held by any given practitioner—such assumptions as the involvement of spiritual entities in healing, delight in sensuality, and a belief in the basic virtues of all healing systems (Mattson 1982: 12). These assumptions are not universal, however, but particular; they bind together subsystems within holistic health. Reichians may reject spiritual entities, but embrace sensuality. Polarity therapists may promote the former, but define the latter as impure.

In the holistic health paradigm, all illness comes from a disturbance in life-force. This force is constructive, mutable, and operates intelligently (Vithoulkas 1981: 26). This is variously expressed as *prana, c'hi*[1], *elan vital,* odic force, orgone energy, or aura and is a blend of the concepts of spirituality and electrical energy. Unless a therapy can affect this force, it produces only superficial change. Awareness of the "tingle" of this force is a basic technique in holistic health practice.

Energy can influence energy (see Mattson 1982: 22). Only another "energy being" (the healer) or a technique that affects the "energy

[1]The romanization of Chinese words is done according to the Wade-Giles system in accordance with older literature.

FIGURE 2.1 ASSUMPTIONS, GOALS, DIAGNOSTIC AND THERAPY CATEGORIES

ASSUMPTIONS

1. The body is the material shadow of energy. This energy may be called chi, prana, odic force, orgone energy or aura and is a blend of the concepts of spirituality and electrical energy. Unless a therapy can affect this force, it produces only superficial change.
2. Energy can affect energy. Only another energy being (the healer) or a technique that affects the energy body (acupuncture, homeopathy) can be effective.
3. Each person is a microcosm of the macrocosm. To understand the individual one must understand the forces and elements of the cosmos. Each person reflects the social environment as well. Thus, personal health and social fulfillment connect intimately. Sickness is a blow to individual and social freedom.
4. Each individual is a unique blend of physical, social, and spiritual forces. Generalization, characteristic of cosmopolitan medicine, is inappropriate.
5. Illness is a lesson. It is a sign that the person is not being used properly. Illness will be either a prelude to a new life-way, if the lesson is learned, or it will be repeated.
6. Physical, emotional, mental, and spiritual realities are inseparably linked. They are interconnected. The most powerful therapies act on the "weak," high-level spiritual sphere.

GOALS

1. Holistic health explicitly seeks to achieve harmony between the forces of the system by changing behavior and engaging the natural defenses of the system.
2. Holistic healers also desire to reintroduce spirituality and empathic sharing into the client-healer relationship.
3. Holistic healers must define themselves distinctly enough to form an economically competitive niche vis-à-vis the orthodox medical community.

DIAGNOSTIC PROCEDURES

1. Assumption: Any part of the body is the microcosm (almost holgraphic) of the whole being and expresses the energetic condition of the body.
   Examples: Iridology, pulse diagnosis, personology, muscle testing, aura analysis
2. Assumption: Body and mind are linked. Behavioral and symbolic cues will provide the basis for understanding the body.
   Examples: Dream interpretation, oral questions, observation of affective state

FIGURE 2.1 (continued)

THERAPIES*

PHYSICAL INTERVENTIONS: Acupuncture, Acupressure, Touch for Health, Jin Shin Do, Electro-acupuncture, Polarity, Neo-Reichian release, Chiropractic, Rolfing, Heat therapies

DIET AND CHEMISTRY: Herbology, Polarity, Naturopathy, Fasting, vitamin therapy, Natural Hygiene, whole food

DIRECT ENERGETIC INTERVENTION: Homeopathy, Psychic healing, Innovative psychology

SELF-EXERCISE THERAPIES: Yoga, Alexander technique, Dance therapy, T'ai Chi, aerobics, polar energetics

*Note: Categories are not mutually exclusive

body" can be effective. Acupuncture, homeopathy, and the laying on of hands are the primary methods of stimulating energy directly. Other techniques are reputed to be less direct.

Each person is a microcosm of the macrocosm. To understand the individual one must understand the forces and elements of the cosmos. Each person reflects the social environment as well. Personal health and social harmony connect intimately. Sickness is a blow to individual and social freedom (Molgaard 1979: 129). In the same vein, each component of the body is a microcosm of the whole body/mind/spirit. This concept is fundamental to the diagnostic and therapeutic techniques that intend to influence an inaccessible organ, such as the liver, by working on its "reflection" or reflex elsewhere on the body. Manipulating points on the hands and feet is part of the practice of reflexology.

The uniqueness of the individual is another major epistemological foundation. Each individual is a unique blend of spiritual, social, environmental, and hereditary forces. Generalizing any characteristic is illegitimate in this system of thought. No head cold is like any other, for the individuals involved are not identical. Factors considered irrelevant in allopathic medicine—for example, the client's favorite color or food—might be crucial in defining each client's unique gestalt. Preferences for cold food might indicate emotional stress in homeopathy, while this is perceived as irrelevant in allopathic medicine.

Illness is no random event in holistic health; it is a lesson. It is a sign that the body and mind are not being used properly. The client's responsibility, with the help of the practitioner, is to determine the nature of the lesson and act accordingly. If the lesson is learned, the illness is a prelude to new life paths. If ignored, the lesson will be repeated, perhaps in a more dramatic way (Bailey 1980: 2–3; Gordon 1981: 24; Mattson 1982: 11). In other words, the cold may be telling the client to slow down or stop eating dairy products and meat. If that is not done, the cold may be suppressed by patent medicines, but it will return as a more hideous illness until the lesson is learned.

Physical, emotional, mental, and spiritual realities are inseparably linked in holistic health. They are nested and interconnected. The physical is the least significant of the subsystems, and only seems important because of its closeness to our perceptions. In holistic health, the most powerful therapies use the least visible, high-level spheres of mind and spirit. Only the agents that act directly on this spirit body, especially homeopathy, acupuncture, and psychic healing, are considered to achieve a long-lasting "cure." The rest are processual measures, part of a long road to well-being. A good bodywork session may incrementally improve the client, but it does not create the fundamental change of spiritual healing.

Holistic health techniques have been developed or borrowed from folk or non-Western traditions that are consistent with these assumptions. These techniques are used with common goals in mind. Holistic health practitioners explicitly seek to achieve harmony on spiritual, social, and personal levels by changing behavior and engaging the natural defenses of the system. Holistic healers actively attempt to reintroduce spirituality and empathic sharing into the client/healer relationship. Educating clients to accept responsibility for their own health care and the prevention of disharmony are the paramount goals (Deliman and Smolowe 1982: 6; Gordon 1981: 17–26; Mattson 1982: 37; Pelletier 1977: 303). A brief scenario, a composite of field experiences, illustrates these concepts.

Peter approaches the office of a holistic health practitioner, Jane, for the first time. Her office is modest, a set of two rooms, located in a small professional building in an older part of Paraiso. The building also contains a chiropractor, a dentist, a psychologist, a physical therapist, and a few physicians. Peter enters the office and is immediately greeted by Jane. She mentions she received the call from his lady, one of her most reliable and enthusiastic clients. Peter is unsure of the situation. Jane is clearly not an M.D. She wears no lab coat, she has no receptionist. She does not even look hurried. In fact, she looks much like his girlfriend. She politely inquires if the appointment is at a good time for him. He responds that it was the *only* time, and he is grateful that she could see him on such short notice. Embarrassed, he admits to feeling terrible. She suggests that they go into the therapy room and discuss it.

They enter a small room with an antique secretary, a wooden massage table, and an oriental chest with many tiny drawers. Against the far wall is a bookshelf, packed with books in varying conditions of newness, volumes on Chinese, Indian, and historical European healing. Another shelf contains paperbacks on psychology, especially Jungian and humanistic, and ethnographies of healing among Native Americans. There are also books on new physics, electronics, and electrical theory. On the secretary are leather bound books entitled *P.D.R. The People's Desk Reference* (an herbal alternative to the *Physician's Desk Reference*), *School of Natural Healing, A Barefoot Doctor's Manual, Jin Shin Do* and a slightly tattered copy of *Touch for Health.* The walls are decorated in Chinese prints and charts of acupuncture meridians, anatomy, and a chart mysteriously labeled "The Law of 5 Elements," containing a five-pointed star and references to numbers and pulses. Jane sits on a swivel chair, motions for Peter to sit on the massage table, and waits for him to speak.

In an increasingly agitated tone, he tells her, "I'm sure Mary told you I am a graduate student . . . I've been feeling like my body is made of bricks, bricks that hurt! I can't sleep. I have all sorts of deadlines, and now I'm catching a cold . . . I can barely sit in a chair, my back hurts so . . . I'm really afraid I just can't make it like this."

Jane nods. She indicates that she understands, after all it was only five years ago that she was getting her master's in psychology. She pauses. While she is sure Mary has described her work, she must make sure that Peter understands what it is that she does. She emphatically states that she cannot fix his body, only he can make those changes. They must cooperate as partners. Before she begins, she must know what he expects her to do, what he thinks she can do.

He grins, sheepishly, and says he wants to remember what it was like to be relaxed. His girlfriend says she gives a great massage. He reflects for half a minute, and adds that he wants to know what is happening to "his body," the body that used to be so healthy. Jane wants to know what feels different to him now.

"I have no energy, I can't sleep. I get angry at little things. All the clinic tells me to do is take two aspirin and go to bed. Jeez! To Bed! How can I go to bed when I have work to do!"

Jane leans forward. "Peter, this is important. What I do is very, very different from an M.D., an allopathic doctor. There is a real difference in what we do in holistic health. In what we do, and how we look at things, I won't claim to cure you. I can help you be more aware of your person . . . your body, your feelings, what you want to have happen. I can't tell you what is wrong with you. Maybe, nothing is wrong . . . you may need to hear what your body is telling you, or else why would it be shouting at you this way? But if you want a grocery list of nasty diseases, I cannot provide that. I can't give you cures, drugs or otherwise. I can tell what you might do to change your diet, your lifestyle . . . get you some tonic herbs . . . I can let you know what your body is telling me. Mary's right too, I can give you a dynamite massage and make you feel better, here and now. Stimulate the ol' lymphatic and circulatory system and move some energy as well. Is that what you want?"

"Yes!"

She tells him to lay down on the table. He shyly asks if it is necessary to remove his clothes. She says that it is not at all necessary in this technique of massage, a combination of Asian practices and reflexology. His back to the table, she begins to hold his face, slowly stroking his forehead and increasing pressure. After he begins to relax, she begins to talk softly.

"I really want you to understand your own body. After you leave here in about an hour and a half, you can say, 'Boy, that woman is sure weird.' You can also act on some of my suggestions and see how they work for you. You see, I can say with some surety, 'This moves energy.' I can't say that what works for Mary will work in the same way for you. That place on your body may plug into something that happened to you fifteen years ago. It may be exactly what you need. We'll have to do it and find out. You are unique. No body out there has your genes, your temperament, your environment, your problems. Whatever has you out of 'sync' has to be rebalanced, or you won't get better. It is as simple as that. But, it isn't easy, it may mean making changes . . . That is your choice, your homework. You may even feel worse, getting better."

Peter grunts out a question. The last concept has perplexed him. He opens his eyes in obvious confusion. He mumbles something that sounds vaguely like 'You mean I'm paying thirty dollars to feel worse?'

Jane smiles. "I really shouldn't put it that way, but I do love people's reactions. What I am saying, is that cup of coffee you had this morning, the crummy feeling you had fifteen years ago, when that foxy girl giggled when you asked her for a date, didn't go away. Before you can be truly well, that has to be dumped. If you hang onto trash at any level, it *will* come back to you. This is really where I differ from an M.D. I'm not going to get rid of your symptoms by suppressing them. I don't want your cold coming back to haunt you as bronchitis, just because you couldn't get rid of the garbage, of whatever kind, that led to it. You just may get that cold you've started, but once it is done . . . It will be gone. Can you accept that?"

Peter is obviously not thrilled. A few minutes of silence later, he lets her know that he does understand her reasoning. He just doesn't want to get sick right now. Jane has seen this problem before. She has even lived it herself! So she makes a contract with him. She lets him know it is his choice. If this is truly not the time to "dump his trash" and live with the consequences, so be it. He is free to pursue the techniques of allopathic medicine, this time. He should also seriously think about coming back to work on it again. He must be honest with himself. Does he want to have a continuous string of annoying illnesses, or is he willing to make a commitment to health, even though it may mean some pain? She goes on to explain that she is oriented primarily toward Chinese medicine. She believes their philosophy is that the path to health is long, but it should not be too traumatic. She ponders to herself that all her peers would not agree. She remembers her own, occasionally torturous road to well-being. She was once impatient to be rid of all her impurities and imbalances immediately! Yet, her own desire for health made her impatient with every episode of "elimination." Years of experience as a practitioner, as well as a client, have shown her a whole spectrum of choices.

After helping him turn over, she continues to work, rhythmically pressing and kneading, occasionally leaning in, using her elbows on a particularly tight spot. He grunts in response to the peculiar mixture of pleasure and pain. She feels it is time to teach about what she is doing.

She tells him that even though he is the only one who knows how his body feels, she can also learn from it. The way he is lying tells her what hurts. She rocks him, noticing which parts move and what parts inhibit the motion. She tells him there are many kinds of bodywork. She initially chose oriental techniques for several reasons. She likes the techniques and is comfortable with them. She feels they are powerful, both relaxing and effective in manipulating energy. She points out that when he first came in, he said he was afraid, and that he had problems with his breathing and with his sleeping. He was also angry. In Chinese medicine, these factors mean something. They are linked together, in cycles of change, the *ko* and *sheng* cycles defining the interaction of the five elementary principles. The Chinese used these cycles to organize their observations. She sees a pattern emerging. She wanted to use that particular set of massage techniques to "test" those patterns. Places of pain and tension, warmth and coolness are used to confirm or reject suspect imbalanced meridians, the channels of the different kinds of energy. Once these are isolated, they can be balanced. The techniques also act as a tonic, balancing all the meridians as the bodywork progresses.

She continues to work in patterns along the back of his body. She asks him questions about his diet, exercise patterns, family, friends, hopes in his given career, and frequently about his fears. She once again turns him over on his back, going back to the face and neck. She "works" on two points for long minutes, them moves on to two other points. By this time, Peter is very relaxed, and soon is snoring softly. Jane leaves him, washes her hands, and then awakens him.

"How are you doing? Don't fall off the table."

She waits until he is fully conscious. He looks at her expectantly and asks what she has learned. She believes she has detected an imbalance in his "kidney meridian." This has little to do with his kidneys per se, more to do with adrenal function. She explains that the Chinese believed that awareness, the capacity to fight for one's goals, almost one's "will", is based on "kidney fire." If that is abused with coffee, stress, fear, and anxiety, then other systems, respiration, digestion, sleep, and the capacity for anger will be affected. Fear is especially symptomatic. She advises him to go home and think about his fear, turning it from anxiety into awareness. She lets him know that he is welcome to contact her any time if he feels distressed. She goes on to suggest that he should cut down on alcohol and coffee. She recommends, making it clear she is not prescribing, tonic herbs. These herbs, she informs him, were what the old Taoist monks used as a balancing formula for the "kidney fire," more like food or vitamins than medicine. She shows him some simple stretching postures to help his lower back. They chat for a few minutes. He writes a check and hands it to her with hug. She suggests that they get together again and gives him some homework. If he is willing, he could make a list of places he feels safe and places he is afraid. They could go over it, and she could try some more intense bodywork techniques. Peter, looking peaceful and slightly intoxicated, walks away.

ROLES AND COMMUNITY
ORGANIZATION

Jane is only a composite. No two practitioners are alike. The diversity within the holistic health community is great. Holistic health community dynamics are based on the roles individuals play in socialization and the creation of the profession. To understand this process, it is necessary to define the kinds of roles and relationships holistic health practitioners create within the geographic community. Socializing new practitioners and educating the community create primary roles around which practitioners cluster. Leaders of resource centers and the "evangelical" creators of various specific therapies form the mobile cores of the holistic health community. Their presence gives a structure to novices and unaffiliated practitioners who would otherwise be on their own. Because there are no strong professional organizations, these ad hoc leaders and culture heroes are the only source of professional exchanges of information, particularly for those "underground" practitioners. For example, Patrick, the leader of a local academy, invites major teachers and practitioners to run workshops at his academy. Novices and holistic health practitioners attend. At these workshops, new skills are acquired and professionalism is instilled.

In addition, professional hierarchies influence a practitioner's relationship to his/her community. An unlicensed massage technician does not interact with the community as obviously or openly as a politically active chiropractor. The constraints and potentials are different and will play an important part in defining the future of a social movement. If holistic health practitioners are to become socially acceptable professionals, members of the community must work together toward that goal. It becomes clear, however, that within the holistic health community not every member can or will choose to make professionalization the primary goal.

Paraiso is a unique community, well-suited for the practice of holistic health and the training of healers. Paraiso is not a solitary community. It sits next to Tierra Buena (population nearly 68,000), a cluster of suburban tracts, farms, and research and development firms. On the other side, lies Agua de Fuente (population only 3,500), haven of the wealthy and important in the history of Paraiso as a once flourishing health resort in the last century. Paraiso itself is a small city, with a population of nearly 75,000. The greater metropolitan area, within the sphere of the study, has only over 100,000 people (Bureau of the Census 1980). No village, it still retains a coastal Californian, provincial atmosphere. Personal growth, research and development, pagan and tourist fiestas, retirement homes, and student hovels exist side by side.

Despite enclaves of Asians, Chicanos and Native Americans, and small pockets of European ethnic groups, the town gives a remarkable appearance of ethnic homogeneity. This is reflected in the census figures for 1980. In Paraiso, Tierra Buena, and Agua de Fuente the population is over two-thirds white, 10 percent Hispanic, with only 2 percent black, 2 percent Asian and nearly 1 percent Native American. Thirty percent of the population has completed one to four years of college. The area is dominated by the tastes of white, upper middle-class bourgeoisie. This is the dominant cultural milieu for holistic health practitioners as well (Mattson 1982: 106). In Paraiso, however, there is also diversity. It stems from subcultural variation. The traditional ethos of Paraiso is tolerance. There are the "street people," resident vagabonds, populating the areas near the beach and in the university student ghetto. Millionaires cluster at the higher elevations. Avocado "ranchers" and research physicists share the sister communities of Paraiso.

A nearby beach village was founded in 1883 as a national Spiritualist center, a permanent camp meeting ground. It grew until oil dominated the scene at the turn of the century (Lathim and Lathim 1975). An hour away, Camino Robles housed a major Theosophical center (Hine 1983: 57). It moved to the area in 1924 and is still a rallying point for esoteric activities. More recently, a messianic community grew and moved on, creating a small health food empire on the way.

Refugees from Los Angeles come seeking "the good life," while, in reverse, others make the easy drive to leave the relaxed, and for them, dull atmosphere of Paraiso. The Mediterranean climate is legendary, and an enduring source of conversation. The greater community seldom harrasses the many cotton-clothed, spiritual residents and even the Safeway stores sell carob milk. The countercultural community, a strong reminder of the politically and socially active sixties, perceives Paraiso as a unique source of healing energy.

Within this context, the holistic health community flourishes. Proximity to Los Angeles, and Camino Robles, connections to the Bay Area and even the San Jaoquin Valley, place Paraiso in a unique position. There is an affluent potential clientele and Paraiso is within commuting distance of the alternative healing centers of Los Angeles and the spiritual centers of Camino Robles. The social climate is not hostile but rather supportive. Health food restaurants, imported natural clothing boutiques, alternative new age craft stores, exercise centers, self-help groups, and county clinics favor the new age lifestyle. Unity, the Unitarians, Church of Religious Science, and various New Thought and more traditional churches lend to the atmosphere of health seeking. As demonstrated in chapter 4, this is no new pattern in Southern California. One local weekly newspaper devotes a section of each issue to spiritual and holistic health activities. In fact, that publication became a major field work resource. Several local "people's handbooks" were written directories for new age activities and holistic health practitioners.

Holistic health practitioners are not a monolithic block. Besides diverse personalities and practices, there is variety of functional roles. A few visiting and local practitioners are renowned catalysts, founders of well-known therapies. Most holistic healers who are visible to the public are practitioners who are also teachers. Some rarely or never teach and prefer to just practice. Among this category are those who choose to work in informal, confidential networks. They may, or may not, choose to practice with the blessing of the law. Novice practitioners, not yet through their rites of passage, may also have informal networks of clients. Of course, no economic community can function without the market that permits these people to explore alternative healing and still pay their rent. At the base of the "practitioner chain" is the client.

Clients use public and private networks to find a practitioner, seeking a "good massage," or an alternative to local physicians. Like the hypothetical Peter, however, clients and practitioners find each other through verbal, interpersonal recommendations. Some clients are "regulars," going as often as once a week. Others go once or twice and then try another practitioner. Documenting this pattern is nearly impossible; most interactions occur sub-rosa. The practitioners may prefer informal conditions, and a greater choice in who will be taken as a client.

Some clientele are deeply influenced by the therapy, others primarily curious. In either case, clients can go out into the community and become novices, the liminal stage between client and practitioner. The options abound. There is one school in which a student can be certified for a unique Paraiso business license, a holistic health practitioner. It also offers credentials in massage and hypnosis and gives credit for the continuing education of nurses. A different school also trains massage technicians and therapists. There is another school for acupuncturists. Workshops are offered through the local adult education facility at the community college, university extension education, the Young Men's Christian Association, herbal stores, the Taoist Sanctuary, the local Zendo, the Yogic Institute/ ashram, and through the churches and independent church/health organizations such as the Polarity Alive Fellowship. Even the local botanical museum offers courses in herbal lore. In addition, the education of a practitioner can be part of an apprentice system, outside any formal insititution. This is all within Paraiso. Beyond the thirty-six locations for learning holistic health in the community, there are seven more in Camino Robles. Five of those are in spiritual growth and psychic healing. Four institutes were frequented in Los Angeles by my informants and eight more throughout the state. A potential practitioner does not lack for choices.

Workshops and lectures provide a forum for holistic health practitioner networking. If Judith Aston's student has a lecture/workshop, she not only draws the Aston Patterners and Rolfers, but Reichians, Rebirthers, Touch for Health practitioners, massage teachers, novices, and potential clients from throughout the community. They meet at the community college on a weekly basis, learning the principles and techniques of movement and posture therapy. More important, they create ties and exchange knowledge. Later at a Neo-Reichian workshop, those ties are reinforced. In a community where the majority of the practices function in small, private, self-contained networks, this interchange is critical in creating the *communitas* of the movement.

Once the decision is made to stand over the table instead of being on it, other decisions need to be made. Practitioner networks may be highly individualized. Practitioners may associate primarily with their clients and a few select friends and colleagues. Communal living is a possibility chosen by some. The Polarity Alive Fellowship and the Society of Emissaries practice jointly tenented "holistic living."

The extent to which an individual wants to practice openly is a critical decision. Advertising requires open, legal, fully documented practitioners. It brings in new clients and it also brings in troublesome ones. Especially in bodywork, these strangers may neither respect nor care about the practitioner's personal and professional integrity. Moreover, expensive and humiliating licensing procedures make overt practice less attractive. Novices trade horror stories of having to be treated "like a prostitute" at the appropriate law enforcement agency that licenses masseuses. In short, many fully socialized and certified practitioners choose to remain in small, intimate networks. They know their clients, and do not have such extensive networks that they must worry about bureaucracy.

Naturally, anyone who uses holistic health as a business, teaches, or advertises must do so publicly and overtly. Qualifications must be clearly visible and consistent with the local governmental regulations. Outside the highly professionalized physicians, chiropractors, dentists, optometrists, psychologists, and acupuncturists, each local city, county, and town sets its own standards for the holistic health practitioner. These must be met. There are exceptions which have clearly had an impact on the development of the field. Religious practices and educational settings are exempt from the issue of practicing medicine without a license. One does not need a license to "teach" bodywork or practice one's religion. It is, therefore, no suprise that some therapeutic groups are also churches and that the workshop format abounds.

In addition, Paraiso is not a closed system. Novices drift into the community to worship the sun and take advantage of the thirty-six resource and educational centers. Once they are trained, they leave for Los Angeles, Seattle, and Nepal. Catalytic figures and teachers are also highly mobile. Nine such prominent figures visited during the period of this study. Especially those in the area of nutrition, psychic healing, and innovative psychology drift in and out of town. This factor has made an accurate census difficult to obtain. Assuming that holistic health practitioners in Paraiso, however short their stay, practice and influence the community, I considered any public display of work between October 1979 and December 1982 for the study. This included advertisements, fliers, newsletters, and assorted publications. In addition, a network of novice and lay practitioners was asked about their professional choices. Analyses of the census and observational data came up with a few patterns illustrative of the factors involved in professional choice.

A discrepancy between the number of people practicing publicly, 253, and the number I knew to be practicing led me to question my census figures. I intuitively knew that something was not right. I knew there was a large population of people practicing confidentially. Although a precise figure is not available, I knew that 800 to 900 people had been trained as massage technicians in Paraiso since 1975, yet only 108 bodyworkers were advertising in any form. What variables were influencing the decision not to practice officially? Could professional status and commitment influence the choice to openly professionalize?

I reorganized my observations to reflect professional status. Clearly, members of what the sociologists call "full," "limited," or "marginal" professionals (Maykovich 1980: 267–69) would each be in a separate category. Characterized by a strong professional identity, organization, lengthy and difficult training period, and autonomy, allopathic medical doctors provide the sociological standard for the "full" professional. The degree of commitment to the field is powerful, and such professionals are unlikely—and often unable—to practice sub-rosa. Presumably, even an M.D. with a holistic health orientation does not lose his valued status. The "limited" professionals include allied health professionals, dentists, psychologists, and optometrists. Limited in what they can do, the specialists lack the autonomy and sanctioned jurisdiction to practice on the entire human body, but they are also highly professionalized. The practitioners who lack the sanction of the American Medical Association are denoted "marginal professionals" (Maykovich 1980: 303). This includes chiropractors and acupuncturists. These practitioners must comply with state regulations, nonetheless; they form professional organizations and are, in California, legally entitled to deliver primary care. Learning and financial commitments are substantially greater than other less regulated holistic health practitioners. Four years of specific professional training are required for chiropractors, at least two for acupuncturists. In California, even archaic evidence demonstarted that 78 percent of graduating chiropractors practiced and 90 percent of those chiropractors practiced in the public eye (Stanford Research Institute 1960: 22, 61). The legal and social forces acting on this category were different from the factors acting on other holistic health practitioners.

I had observed that people who intended to be technicians or permanent novices/workshop addicts seldom planned to practice overtly. I must emphasize that this does not mean the holistic health practitioners and technicians are evading legal requirements, only that they practiced in private, confidential networks. A business license does not necessarily mean an individual practices outside the intimate sphere of known clients. Only 8 percent of the technicians and novices I knew went on to practice publicly, while 30 percent of those committed to a greater range of therapies, and professional identity—holistic health practitioners—became openly acknowledged practitioners. This is similar to the proportion of Ayurvedic practitioners registered in India. There, too, one third practices overtly and officially (Leslie: 1975: 407). Brown-Keister's study of holistic health practitioners in the Bay Area produced a similar figure of 40 percent (Mattson 1982: 106). Given this spread, I wanted to know if the educational and professional difference was a significant one.

It appeared that practitioners and technicians made different choices about the degree of public exposure they would adopt in their practices. This makes sense, given that becoming a licensed "holistic health practitioner" takes twice as much money and time as it does to become a technician. Licensing involves a straightforward demonstration of education, certification, and the purchase of a business license. However, massage technicians and those still in the process of learning must be licensed through law enforcement agencies. In the minds of the bureaucracy, bodywork and prostitution are inexorably linked. Moreover, the very ambiguity of the role of "bodyworker" produces an unpredictable clientele. Is massage a therapy or a vice? The practice of "Ayurvedic medicine" is more clearly "therapeutic" than "massage," which is occasionally a euphemism for prostitution in the public lexicon. Hoping to escape this stereotype, the massage community promotes "ethical massage." The image persists, however.

Once I understood there were three separate professional communities, with different proportions of confidential practitioners, I needed to address the next question. I knew about the tip of the iceberg, the overt practitioners, but I did not know how many sub-rosa practitioners were out there, quietly practicing, exchanging massages and information. I knew approximately how many public practitioners were in each category. Using simple algebra, I could estimate the number of sub-rosa practitioners using my known parameter and my statistical proportions (see Palumbo 1977: 280–84). This allowed me to deduce that there are probably approximately 360 privately active holistic health practitioners and 200 massage technicians and novices. In all three categories—professional, holistic health practitioner, and technician—I estimated a population of approximately 790 to 830 practicing holistic healers in the immediate community. This reflects the intuitive estimation that at least that many bodywork therapists had been trained to practice in Paraiso, and there are even more in other categories of holistic health.

In summary, holistic health practitioners possess a solidly consistent set of assumptions, the only uniformity in the population. There is variation in the choice of lifestyles and professional goals. An individual can live a private life, practicing among close friends and peers. Communal living and intensive community involvement are also well within the choices. Commitment to an established profession is possible, as well as commitment to establishing a profession. These are organizational variables that define the practitioners of Paraiso. In addition, holistic health is highly diverse, and the symbolic content of the practice creates nominal categories—bodyworker, psychic healer, Touch for Health practitioner, and so forth—that define the community. Organization and context both play a part in shaping the holistic health movement.

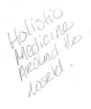
Holistic Medicine Around the World.

HOLISTIC HEALTH THERAPIES

It is with their muscles that they most easily obtain knowledge of the divine. (*Ends and Means*, Huxley 1969: 235)

In the previous chapter I was able to analyse the organization of the holistic community. There are also other ways of acquiring a descriptive understanding. In writing about the Azande, Evans-Pritchard contended that their system of magic was logical, given its own premises. The components of their world view were interdependent and internally consistent (1964: 98–99). The major deviation from "European" thinking was not in the quality of the logic, but in the premises. Magic proceeded from different assumptions and so created a disparate conceptual reality. Similarly, the naturalistic medical traditions of the Old World—Asian, Ayurvedic, and Hippocratic medicine—and the syntheses of holistic health, are logically consistent paradigms, given their unique postulates. By looking at the various lines of reasoning, and the derivative techniques, I seek to illustrate the logical uniformity, as well as the diversity of detail.

Each holistic health practitioner is defined within his/her community by several variables. The nature of the "practice" is a primary defining factor. To understand the diverse systems of medical belief and practice, it is useful to consider the immense variation within the holistic health community. The different kinds of medical beliefs often reflect the geographical and historical development of these practices. For example, there are obvious philosophical and practical similarities among Asian based practices, distinct from techniques derived from the Hippocratic tradition or from modern humanistic psychology.

It has already been mentioned that holistic health practitioners hold certain assumptions in common. This includes a belief in vital energy as a primary explanatory model. Holism—the perception that spirit, mind, and body are inseparably linked—is basic. It is holistic health, after all. The dominance of spirit and mind are also clearly articulated. No body is truly distinct and separate from the universe but is a microcosm. Yet, no body is like any other. Each is unique. Out of these assumptions grow a variety of diagnostic and therapeutic beliefs and practices.

The varieties of holistic health, East Asian, Indian, European/Arabic medicine, and modern psychological and religious practices reflect this. All have clearly created a synthesis made up of American culture and a parent tradition. East Asian medicine refers to a set of beliefs derived from China, Japan, and Korea but practiced in Southern California, as understood by Americans. These are not cross-cultural practices as much as cross-cultural composites. Unfamiliar beliefs are interpreted through familiar values. In this section, I will examine and discuss each category. This includes defining the range of practices under each category—assumptions, etiology, diagnostic and therapeutic concepts. The latter might well include both tonic/preventative and "curative" strategies. To illustrate the diversity of techniques under the rubric, holistic health, I will demonstrate how each would cope with a common syndrome, a headache.

ASIAN BASED THERAPIES

There is an impressive range of therapies that use assumptions and techniques derived from East Asian medicine. Some practices are truly cross-cultural imports. The individuals in such practices are practitioners from Taiwan, Japan, or Korea. They use "pure" forms of acupuncture (using needles to stimulate the acupuncture meridians, see Figure 2.1), moxabustion (the use of burning mugwort, *Artemesia vulgaris* on the meridian points) and tonic and curative herbalism (Academy of Traditional Chinese Medicine 1975: 28–29). The traditional practices themselves are not homogenous. Family practices, spanning some generations, may use specific techniques that are not widely shared. In addition, experimentation in Europe, the People's Republic, Taiwan, and Japan has produced a revised numbering and associative system for the meridians. The traditional meridians are said to flow in a specific direction, beginning at a set point and ending at a certain point. This system has been revised. These revisions are reflected in the current training of Asian acupuncturists.

Of course, there are also wide regional variations in practice and style. Most of these variations are known within Paraiso by reputation only. There is only one openly practicing Chinese acupuncturist and a variety of "unofficial," small scale medical entrepreneurs. It is believed, nonetheless, that Japanese acupuncturists using *kanpo* (Chinese medicine) may not use the same classical techniques retained by a Chinese acupuncturist. In addition, regional variations in China are reputed to be pronounced. Korean acupuncturists are reknowned for the use of long, slender needles and are believed, by the holistic health community, to still retain an association with Taoist mysticism and traditional shamanism.

Asian-American or Asian practitioners are only the tip of the iceberg. The overwhelming majority of the practitioners of traditional Asian medicine are Euro-American students who are two or three student generations removed from the original Asian therapist. They may use classical techniques, often jointly with martial arts or an Asian/American religion. Synthesists may also use a modern offshoot, electro-acupuncture, Touch for Health, and acupressure in its various permutations, shiatsu, *tsubo, jin shin do, jin shin jyutsu, do-in* and *g-jo.*

Whatever the variations, the techniques mentioned are based on a set of common assumptions. They all acknowledge the basic premise that energy flow is the basis of organic function (see Figure 3.1). This energy is a pervasive environmental constant. It is absorbed into living entities and is the vital force. In human beings the energy enters through food (*ku ch'i*) and breath (*ta ch'i*) and is ultimately transformed into *chen ch'i.* Chen ch'i nourishes and defends the body and provides for reproduction (Teeguarden and Teeguarden 1978b: 9). The ch'i travels along paths of "least resistance" in the body. Each of these "energy freeways" is a meridian and each is named after an organ in the human body. This is misleading, however. Each meridian is associated with an organ function in the body (Porkert 1980: 106; 164–5; Revolutionary Health Committee of Hunan 1977: x; Teeguarden and Teeguarden

FIGURE 3.1 FUNDAMENTALS OF ASIAN MEDICINE

Diagnosis and treatment are based on the manipulation of energy, *ch'i,* as it passes through specific channels, the meridians. The meridians are organized by functional elements, and structured by the degree of yin/yang. Each channel governs a particular set of bodily functions. Each meridian is paired with another of the same element [Note: FIRE has four meridians]. Yin meridians are always paired with yang. The meridians interact with each other according to the relationships defined by "The law of the five elements."

THE YIN/YANG RHYTHM CONTINUUM

YIN	ABSOLUTE YIN	LESSER YIN	GREATER YIN	LESSER YANG	SUNLIGHT YANG	GREATER YANG	YANG
	chueh-yin	*shao-yin*	*t'ai-yin*	*shao-yang*	*yang-ping*	*t'ai-yang*	

ACUPUNCTURE MERIDIANS

ELEMENT	EMOTION	YIN/YANG	MERIDIAN FUNCTION	ENERGETIC FUNCTION
FIRE	Mania/Joy	Lesser yin	Heart	Seat of "Spirit" (shen)
		Greater yang	Small Intestines	Assimilation, temporary energy storage
		Absolute yin	Pericardium—Circulation/Sex	Source of pleasure
		Lesser yang	Triple Heater (respiration, digestion, excretion)	Circulation of fluids and postnatal ch'i
EARTH	Worry/Sympathy	Sunlight yang	Stomach	Controls energy derived from food
		Greater Yin	Spleen/Pancreas	Root of the constitution
METAL	Grief/Release	Greater Yin	Lungs	Absorbs and transforms ch'i from the environment to internal ch'i
		Sunlight Yang	Large Intestine	Transportation and transformation
WATER	Fear/Resolution	Greater Yang	Bladder	Physical protection, completes the Kidney meridian functions
		Lesser Yin	Kidney	Seat of potential energy (chih) the source of ch'i
WOOD	Anger/Will	Lesser Yang	Gall Bladder	Movement of physical energy
		Absolute Yin	Liver	Seat of "Will," and planning

FIGURE 3.1 *(continued)*

THE CYCLES OF THE FIVE ELEMENTS

KO CYCLE of stimulation/ SHENG CYCLE of sedation

FIRE	creates	EARTH,	is inhibited by	WATER,	and inhibits	METAL
EARTH	creates	METAL,	is inhibited by	WOOD,	and inhibits	WATER
METAL	creates	WATER,	is inhibited by	FIRE,	and inhibits	WOOD
WATER	creates	WOOD,	is inhibited by	EARTH,	and inhibits	FIRE
WOOD	creates	FIRE,	is inhibited by	METAL,	and inhibits	EARTH

EXAMPLE: Stimulating the WATER Kidney meridian will
1. stimulate the "husband" WATER Bladder meridian;
2. stimulate the "son," WOOD Liver/Large Intestines meridians;
3. sedate the various FIRE meridians—Heart, Small Intestine, Pericardium, Triple Heater
4. stimulating the EARTH Stomach, or Spleen meridians would sedate the Kidney meridian

(from Academy of Traditional Chinese Medicine 1975; Porkert 1976; 1980; Selinsky n.d.; Teeguarden and Teeguarden 1978; Teeguarden 1980a, Vieth 1972)

1978b: 3). The meridian is not "the kidney," but linked with the renal and adrenal physiological functions as well as specific "energetic" activities.

The energy is defined by two characteristics, its functional elemental nature and a measure of "structural potential," yin/yang (Porkert 1980: 13–14; Teeguarden and Teeguarden 1978a: 2–3). There are five elemental principles: fire, earth, metal, water, wood. Each is associated with color, taste and odour, emotion, sound, season, climate, anatomical focus, and the ability to change a state of being. For example, water is blue, salty, and when out of balance, putrid smelling. It is akin to fear and resolution. It is associated with groaning, winter, and cold. Water governs bones. It is associated with the power to emphasize, not balance or decrease. The presence of any of these variables would indicate the element water. Yin is the most passive state, and therefore is characteristic of storage, of potential. Yang is the active, "full" state. Yang limits yin structural potential. Yang cannot "become full," because it already is all it can be. These two variables, elements and potential, combine to form the meridians.

Along each meridian are various points that are numbered in the direction of energy flow. For example, the beginning of the "kidney" meridian is K1, the point where ch'i enters the body. The end is K27.

Each point is associated with a physiological process. K1, bubbling spring, is indicated in coma, shock, mania, and epilepsy. K27 is associated with chest pain, cough, asthma, and vomiting (Academy of Traditional Chinese Medicine 1975: 154–61; Teeguarden and Teeguarden 1978b: 24–25). Dysfunction is caused by blocks or leakages of ch'i. The goal of the practitioner is to discern the area of difficulty, determine whether it is excess or deficient, and reinstate balance.

Imbalance is the source of disease. Balance, longevity, and clear thinking are the clearly articulated goals of Asian/American medicine. The imbalance may have been brought on by a variety of causes. These include exposure to external forces; temperature, dietary (chemical) and physical stress, social conditions, and injury (Revolutionary Health Committee of Hunan 1977: 25). Asian practitioners also pinpoint internal states. Emotions and attitudes are as responsible for ill health as any environmental factor (Yamamoto 1979: 49). The path to well-being in Asian medicine involves behavioral change. Although that change is initiated by a practitioner, it is ultimately the client's responsibility to achieve balance (1979: 43–44).

Various therapies use the idea of ch'i and the five elements but are different in specific techniques or specializations. For example, shiatsu, derived from *amma* uses rhythmic pressure/percussion massage to stimulate most of the acupuncture points along the twelve "organ" meridians. In America, shiatsu is usually regimented and routinized, focusing on overall tonification. Only a basic knowledge of the meridians is needed to practice shiatsu at the technician level of expertise.

Jin Shin Do, however, is based on slightly different techniques (Teeguarden 1978; Teeguarden and Teeguarden 1978a; 1978b; 1978c). Besides the twelve "organ" meridians, there are the "strange flows," connecting the meridians and acting as governors. These are automatic controls for the organ meridians. There are forty points that can manipulate the strange flows directly. These are the key points in Jin Shin Do. They can be used to release and balance the organ meridians and can specifically focus on therapeutic problems.

Touch for Health is another example demonstrating the diversity of the Asian medical system (Thie 1979). Founded by a chiropractor, this therapy system believes that meridians not only govern a set of physiological functions but also the muscles directly in the area of the flows. The meridians can then be investigated by using muscle testing, a set of techniques designed to determine the response of a particular group of muscles. If one wants to determine the state of the kidney meridian, which runs through the psoas muscle, then one tests the psoas. This is done by having the client lie down with the foot at a forty-five degree angle, slightly to the side with the foot pointing out. Putting pressure on the inside of the foot and pushing slightly down and out, should cause the foot to stay put if the muscle is supported by its meridian. If the leg sags weakly with slight pressure, then the meridian is out of balance. Using the five elements, the origin of the weakness can be determined and acupressure points (as well as other points) can be used to strengthen the meridian (Thie 1979: 64–65). This is an important synthesis, since the weakest point in importing East Asian medicine is the complex skill involved in diagnosis.

Diagnoses in traditional East Asian medicine are based on pulse, observation, inquiry, and the palpation of painful areas. The pulse diagnoses is by far the most sensitive technique and difficult to master. The twelve organ meridians can be detected through pulses, three places on each wrist, at shallow and deep levels. There are at least twenty-eight variables to detect. Threadiness, strength, evenness of flow, and fullness are among the most obvious (Hastings 1981: 468). Decades are needed to fully command pulse reading.

Observing behavior and bodily state can be used to determine both physical and mental/emotional states. Observing the smell, color and texture of skin, tongue, ears, perspiration or urine, and the sounds of voice, breath, or stomach are in the diagnostic repertoire (Chang 1978: 50; Hastings 1981: 468; Revolutionary Health Committee of Hunan 1977: 21). For example, if there are blemishes on the young adolescent skin, where are they? Do they cluster along a specific meridian? If so, then that might be an initial point of inquiry. There is also a complex system of physiognomy, using bodily features to reveal personality. One handy diagnostic tool is determining *sanpaku.* If the area over the iris of the eye is white, then the individual is dangerously, excessively yang. Dangerously, because such an individual might well harbor an unpredictable rage. The gall bladder meridian might be a good place to look for a major imbalance. Similarly, if the white of the eye is showing under the iris, the person is yin sanpaku, hazardously over yin. A kidney imbalance, stemming from excess use of kidney fire (adrenal function), is draining the person's energy and will. Such individuals are prone to accident and despair (Teeguarden 1978: 38–39).

Asking questions is well within the diagnostic tradition of East

Asian medicine. Naturally, there are questions about location, onset, and history of the difficulty. Such pertinent topics as sleep patterns, eating and bowel habits, menstrual and childbirth data are also queried (Kao 1973: 5; Revolutionary Health Committee of Hunan 1977; 19). In addition, there are also pointed inquiries into emotional states and dreams, to reveal symbolism associated with the five elements. Dreams of worms and wounds, shipwrecks, drowning, and incomplete sex indicate an imbalance of the kidney meridian (Teeguarden and Teeguarden 1978c: 10). Groans, fear, and paranoia would also be linked to this meridian.

Therapy is based on manipulation of energy, directed through dietary changes, herbs, physical manipulation, and physical and spiritual exercise. Herbal and dietary changes may be either tonic or curative. Tonic herbs and dietary schemes are the equivalent of preventative medicine. They are designed to improve the overall stamina of the individual, increasing ch'i, longevity, virility, and other appealing characteristics. Each food and herb is associated with one of the five elements, as well as having empirically derived uses (Teeguarden 1980b).

Balance is achieved by manipulating "command points" on the specific meridian, as well as other meridians. Command points are a set of points on either the hand or foot, associated with each of the five elements (Selinsky n.d.). Each element influences the other elements in a specific way (see Figure 3.1). For example, fire is dowsed by water, metal yields water, and water grows wood. Thus to increase the amount of energy in a water associated meridian, one would increase metal, or decrease fire, using either the command points on the kidney meridian or a meridian associated with metal or fire (Teeguarden 1980a). Invoking a command point will increase, decrease, or balance the energetic flow. Using the strange flows—energy flows linking the organ meridian system—also can directly manipulate the balance. Moxa, needles, and finger pressure are traditional methods of manipulation. Electrical stimulation is a modern variation on an ancient theme (Gunji 1973: 42–47).

Attitude change, meditation, and physical/ spiritual exercise are significant tools of holistic therapy. Because of the unity of mind and body in this approach "physical therapies" are intertwined with Taoist, Buddhist, or Confucianist philosophical/meditation centers and martial arts. T'ai chi ch'uan, a martial art, is prescribed as a "meridian tonic" by some acupuncturists.

A culture-specific syndrome provides an example of this behavioral link. There is a proverbial syndrome, "meditator's disease," said to result from overstimulation of the parasympathetic nervous system. In a sense, it is the opposite of the various "stress" syndromes in western societies. Instead of a constant feeling of fight or flight, there is unwavering peace and bliss. There is so little stimulation, that the body can eventually no longer maintain itself. It is a fatal flaw that must be corrected if the body is to survive. One story of a recovery is about Hakuin, the founder of the *Renzai* sect of Zen Buddhism. After repeated negative prognoses, Hakuin was finally accepted as a "client" by a mountain shaman. This shaman re-rooted Hakuin, making him perceive the dynamic balance of the five elements in mundane life. The treatment of his "disease" was behavioral. All aspects of his daily life, including exercise, food, and work were manifestations of the five elements and were employed to cure the legendary Hakuin. A specific medical context was not necessary.

East Asian medicine takes several approaches to the specific problem of a headache. Headache is an ambiguous syndrome and Asian medicine uses many explanations and treatment strategies—there are headaches caused by "liver" and "gall bladder" meridian imbalances. Headaches based on the liver meridian, "toxic" headaches, are associated with insomnia, dry mouth with thin tongue fur, a full liver meridian pulse, exhaustion, and anger. Treatment can include acupuncture, acupressure, and an herbal concoction of gentian, chrysanthemum flowers, gambir, pre-cooked oyster shell, magnetite, hemlock parsley, and self-heal (Revolutionary Health Committee of Hunan 1977: 77–79). The liver meridian is paired with the gall bladder, another suspect for headaches. This kind of headache is accompanied by stiff neck, irritability, fever, perspiration, a bitter taste in the mouth, abdominal swelling, foggy vision, and painful ribs (Teeguarden 1980a: 62; Thie 1979: 88). The diet should be changed to minimize fatty foods. Jin Shin Do treatments would concentrate on releasing the four strange flow points that coincide with the liver and gall bladder meridians (Teeguarden and Teeguarden 1978a: 18). Touch for Health practitioners would trace the gall bladder meridian (touching the length of the meridian with the hand) and hold four points along the gall bladder, stomach, and liver meridians and four "neuro-lymphatic" points on each side of the torso (Thie 1979: 88–89). The latter technique is designed to release the block of energy directing lymph flow (1979: 22), a non-Asian addition to the sequence. Traditional acupuncture and moxabustion treatments of such headaches would easily employ fourteen points along the gall bladder, bladder, stomach, and governing vessel (a strange flow) meridians (Toguchi 1974: 197–98). There are clearly connections between the various approaches, but considerable leeway in the implementation of the therapies.

SYNTHETIC AYURVEDIC PRACTICES

Ayurvedic medicine is India's classical, naturalistic medical system. It has had profound historical influence on the East Asian and Hippocratic traditions, as we shall see in chapter 4. Unlike its East Asian kin, Ayurvedic medicine is rarely practiced in a "culturally pure" form in Paraiso. There is one practitioner of Ayurvedic/Unani medicine, per se, and he is strongly influenced by the concepts of homeopathy. This is not suprising. Ayurvedic practitioners in India coexist successfully with homeopaths (Leslie 1976b; 359–60; Montgomery 1976: 278). Specific practices—such as the ever-popular Yoga—were easily found in Paraiso. At the primary location of my fieldwork, the holistic health practitioner trainees met regularly before instruction began to learn Yoga from an alumnus of the school. Nearby a major Yogic ashram flourished. Yoga was taught in university extension classes, at the YMCA, and as sidelines for a variety of holistic health practitioners.

The influence of Ayurvedic thought on holistic health is primarily through syncratic doctrines. In America, this is especially true for Polarity therapy, and for Arica therapy elsewhere in the Americas and Europe (Green 1981: 101–2). In spite of these variations, the synthetic practices retain many of the basic assumptions of classical Indian medicine. This includes the manipulation of elemental energy, a focus on reincarnation and personal evolution toward a divine state, and to a far lesser degree, the idea of humors or *doshas.* Therapeutically, the basic approaches are similar to the East Asian tradition. Dietary change, massage, and attitude alteration are the keys to recreating balance, the healing goal of Ayurvedic medicine.

Vital force, prana, in imbalance, is the basis of all disease and, flowing properly, is the source of all well-being. As in the East Asian system, life energy is available from the outside environment and is transformed into a suitable form. There are five elements in the

Ayurvedic system as well, although they differ from the Chinese paradigm. Each has a function and a host of associations in taste, color, and spiritual quality, and each is reflected in virtually every physical manifestation. The five *bhutas* are fire, earth, water, air, and ether, the stuff of the cosmos. They are related to digestion, bones and solidity, vital fluids, nervous function, and integration of bodily networks, respectively.

The energy exists on an ethereal plane. Once it enters, it cycles through the body in a series of chakras. These chakras are believed to act on the body by regulating the endocrine system. The chakras are envisioned as nodes of rotating energy, they are associated with the elements, colors, and diverse virtues. Although of theoretical importance in Ayurvedic medicine, they are not the focus of practice. Synthetic systems, however, such as Polarity and Arica center on the chakras and they are critical in psychic healing.

In the traditional Ayurvedic system, the five elements combine to form three humors, the *tridosha:* 1) Phlegm (*kaph*), combining earth and water; 2) Bile (*pitta*), combining earth and fire; and 3) Wind (*vayu*), combining air and ether. The tridosha are the basis of diagnoses and therapy. Body shape, behavior, and symptoms are associated with an excess or deficiency of a particular dosha (Das and Satsang 1978: 53–57; Obeyeskere 1977: 158–59; Sharma 1979: 17–21). Diet, including herbal and mineral treatments, yogic postures and meditation, and physical manipulations are designed to rebalance the humors.

In translation to American culture, the tridosha system is largely bypassed. Rather than combining the elements into humors, the elements themselves are the basis of diagnostic and therapeutic decisions. For example, in the Ayurvedic system, a respiratory cold clearly reflects an excess of phlegm. In the classic Ayurvedic system, this would be the basis of dietary changes—elimination of milk and sweet foods—and the prescription of pungent foods and herbs would follow. Kaph-increasing yogic postures would be eliminated. In the syncretic system, such as Polarity therapy, this would happen implicitly, but not explicitly. Phlegm is a mixture of earth and water elements. Polarity would go directly to the earth and water elements, and do roughly the same "work." The same category of foods would be eliminated, and "polar-energetic" exercises would be assigned. These are postures and movements based loosely on *kundalini* yoga. They are short duration, physically intense postures that are meant to produce the maximum change in minimum time. Especially crucial are squatting/breathing postures designed to open the sacrum—focus of the lower breath. In addition, any imbalance is seen as an expression of lifestyle disharmony. Somewhere in the individual's childhood or recent life history, a "bad" decision was made and a disharmonious concept formed. The person is aided by a Polarity therapist "facilitator" in Gestalt therapy, role playing, and general catharsis. Often simultaneously, this accompanies *tomasic* and *satvik* Polarity therapy.

Traditionally, tomasic, satvik and *rajasic* refers to destructive, balanced, and creative energies or processes. In Polarity, they refer to therapeutic categories based on the idea of dynamic energy. Tomasic therapy is destructive, designed to break up blocks of frozen energy and allow the suppressed physical expression of the emotion to emerge and flow freely. It is characteristically intense and involves deep massage and manipulation. Emotions and pain are meant to flow freely. Screams are permitted if not encouraged. Satvik manipulation and therapy aim at restoring balance after the traumatic tomasic therapy has allowed the energy to flow. Satvik therapy is gentle, two-handed holding and light-touching massage.

Polarity therapy was created by a mystic chiropractor/naturopath, Randolph Stone (1953; 1957; 1978). It is a highly innovative synthesis of Ayurvedic medicine, bodily manipulation, American herbal medicine, and American morality. His therapy split into two distinct schools of thought. One school, based in Southern California, guided by Pierre Pannetier is more "satvik" and oriented toward gentle physical therapy (see Pannetier 1978: 216–18). The other branch of Polarity therapy is based in the Northwest. Orcas Island Polarity centers more on communal lifestyle than simply diet and physical therapy. This faction of Polarity was much more strongly represented in Paraiso during the time of my fieldwork. Under the charismatic leadership of Jefferson Campbell, the Indian moral and religious orientation is more pronounced.

The basic tenets of Ayurvedic medicine are intimately linked with Hinduism. They reflect some of the biases that have evolved hand in hand with the hierarchical social structure of India. Karma, learning to fit into one's inborn place in the scheme of things, is the basis of imbalance and disease (see Bailey 1980: 20). In the classical Indian system, the high status of priests and male human beings in general was reinforced by these ideas. Prayer and theurgy—the use of ritual and meditation to influence the spiritual plane, particularly to enhance spiritual growth—were the highest goals of the medical system. "Semen"—an innate genital secretion possessed by both men and women (although female semen is inferior to male)—is believed to be the most refined fluid, and if misused, a major source of illness (Gandhi 1978: 145; Obeyeskere 1976: 213–15). In translation to Euro-American culture, these basic orientations were kept and given an American flavor. Since American culture lacks priests, "spiritual leaders" are regarded as having the highest status and have the ability to diagnose karmic miscarriage. Inability to learn that familial obligations and the failure of men and women to recognize their gender roles as part of their karmic burden is seen as a major source of imbalance and disease. Celibacy in couples, as practiced by Indian forebearers, is considered a positive virtue. In fact, the purification period in Polarity involves a month of celibacy, and practitioners recommend much longer. Loss of semen and excessive contact with the "negative" energy of women is considered unhealthy for both partners and for any potential offspring.

Astrology plays a part in traditional Ayurvedic medicine and has been added to the diagnostic tools of the Polarity therapists. Although usually the realm of psychic healers, Mediterranean and European astrology is used to diagnose potential "areas of weakness," which can then be manipulated according to Ayurvedic principles. Hippocratic medicine links astrological associations, the houses of the zodiac and the four elements of the Greek tradition—fire, air, water, and earth—with anatomy. For example, air is represented by Aquarius, Gemini, and Libra and is linked to ankles, shoulders, and kidneys/adrenal glands. The presence of certain planets in the various astrological houses hints at possible disfunctions of the various anatomical parts (Garrison 1973; Jones 1978; 163; Stone 1957: 46–54). The process of astrological diagnosis can be complex, and although I never saw it being used as the sole tool, it gives its practitioners a point of inquiry.

Diagnostic procedures are quite similar to the practices of East Asian medicine. Dreams, behavior, the smell and color of bodily excretions, and body type form the basis of diagnostic inquiries. In Polarity, each of the five elements is "reflected" in various areas of human anatomy. For example, each toe is associated with one of the five elements. The big toe is a reflex of ether, the second toe, air, and so forth. Injuries, callouses (it is believed callouses do not develop in areas of balanced energy), or deformities of any kind would indicate an imbalance in energy. Other therapeutic practices could then be invoked. The aesthetic arrangement of food is a function of ether. Eating a burrito slapped on a plate is decidedly deficient in ether. An appreciation of beauty and elegance in eating, personal appearance, and the environment are encouraged.

Much of the Polarity Alive Fellowship lifestyle is directed to chronic karmic improvement and preventative medicine. Each of us, the cosmology reveals, chooses a particular life, drawn to the karmic burden of our parents. "Working through" the errors of past behavior and past lives is the highest duty of an individual. Part of this karmic load is expressed in the body and is linked to the astrological "imprint" of the person's birth. Materially altering the body through physical therapy, as well as improving emotionally and spiritually is the mechanism for this "work." This concept is directly tied to the Hippocratic/naturopathic conceit of "elimination." Implicit in elimination is the idea that nothing ever disappears. A hostile or envious thought, a greasy hamburger, a lie, all stain the karma, and its reflection, the body. To eliminate this taint, the emotion, toxin, or sin must be expelled. The catharsis might well be traumatic. The longer the taint is retained, the more painful the evacuation. Karmic burdens not eliminated during this lifetime are brought to the next, adding to the task of purification. Moreover, karma is intertwined with genetics, so that abusing one's own karma creates a degenerating species. Achieving purity becomes a lifelong and paramount task.

Cleansing as a way of life is the daily routine of the Polarity therapist, and to some extent, his client. Central to the therapy is periodic fasting and the "purifying diet" (Kalson and Kalson 1979: 8). Meat and drugs such as orally consumed caffeine and alcohol are expressly forbidden. Sprouted grains, fresh fruits and vegetables, and their juices are the only acceptable purifying cuisine. Daily doses of "liver flush," a mixture of oil, lemon juice, and garlic are advised. Diuretic, laxative, and expectorant teas are given to help the elimination process. In the throes of deep purification, vomiting is induced and caffeine enemas are given. Any process of bodily discharge, such as diarrhea, colds, or nausea is actually a positive sign of elimination. This was brought home to me one day, when after a few weeks of "purification," I came dragging into a group therapy session, commenting on my overall wretchedness. "Great," was the response, "You are finally getting rid of all that old junk."

Other Ayurvedic therapies are adopted into Polarity practice. *Shivambu kelpa* is a practice used both in this segment of the holistic health community and in many others, involving drinking/recycling of urine, "the water of life." It is explained as a method of recycling the minerals lost by tainted and inefficient bodies. It is also an immediate negative reinforcement for eating meat or using drugs, since these practices are reputed to make the process highly unpalatable. Recognized as a clearly "foreign" therapy, practitioners are sometimes reluctant to recommend it or even to admit to practicing it. One interesting variation of this practice involves making a homeopathic dilution of urine. The urine itself is not consumed, only its energy "shadow," for the urine is so dilute that there may be little physically present.

Polarity, a combination of Ayurvedic and Hippocratic therapy is complex and diverse. One set of therapeutic goals revolves around spiritual and physical purification on a daily and lifelong basis. Another involves acute processes. These illness episodes are justified by the elimination paradigm. To some extent, they must also be eased. No medical system can function without some alleviation of symptoms because the clients will not tolerate it. I will return to our example of a headache. In Polarity therapy, this headache is perceived as an excess of wind in the bloodstream, too much fire and air, or it might result from improper colon cleansing, creating a toxic overload. In either case, there are physical, dietary, and postural/exercise therapies to rely on. Placing the left, or the receptive hand,over the pain, and placing the right hand under the head, balances the energy flow. Fasting and drinking fresh lemon and clover or alfalfa tea is advised to purify the blood (Stone 1978: 13, 50, 64). Finally, a balancing posture, such as a squat, with the feet placed closely together, may be used to open the body. Additional postures may be advised. One technique involves placing the little fingers in the ears, rocking gently in a squat and humming (Stone 1953: 79). Like other therapies derived from the Hippocratic tradition, however, the focus is primarily on chronic, not acute conditions.

EURO-AMERICAN NATURALISTIC MEDICAL SYSTEMS

Asia was hardly the only continent to conceive a naturalistic medical tradition. Hippocratic medicine also focused on elemental energy, the equilibrium of natural and internal forces as the source of well-being. Illness was conceived, once again, as the result of the imbalance of these forces. Much of chapter 4 is devoted to tracing the lines of descent of the complex European medical traditions. The heirs to these traditions thrive in holistic health. A varied assortment of diagnostic and therapeutic techniques have evolved, or been handed down, that are consistent with the basic principles of Hippocratic medicine, especially the empiricist school.

Naturalistic medical systems are rooted in the concept that natural forces in balance will produce health and wholeness. The etiology of illness stems from disharmony among the various natural elements and energies. Ancient Hippocratic lore states that since the forces that cause "dis-ease" are natural, only natural forces can be effective in healing. Modern holistic health practitioners have adopted this philosophy. The impression that nature is ultimately benign and will always promote health is profound and pervasive. "Synthetic" chemicals, clothes, and philosophies lack the vital force, tainting the process of energy flow. This belief generated the methodology of drugless therapy and minimum intervention with body processes.

The foundation of the Hippocratic diagnostic approach is the concept that each anatomical part reflects the whole entity. That being is, in turn, a microcosm of the cosmic macrocosm. This philosophy posits a pervasive "Intelligence," that seeks harmony as its apogee, its highest goal. Illness is perceived as part of an ongoing spiritual evolution, a single episode in the history of the growth or failure of the individual. The concept of "elimination," so fundamental to Polarity therapy, is the base line for naturopathic medicine, homeopathy, and most bodywork (Christopher 1979: 517), as well as natural hygiene—the discipline most recently promoted on a national scale by Harvey and Marilyn Diamond in their book *Fit for Life* (1985).

Homeopathy has taken this concept to its logical conclusion. Philosophically, homeopathy envisions all disease stemming from ancient suppressions of genetic/karmic weaknesses. These "miasms" must be expressed and rebalanced. If not, the species, and certainly the individual will continue to suffer exponentially with each suppression. Hahnemann, the founder of the homeopathic school, used a little known concept in Hippocratic lore. He postulated that the body's innate homeostatic mechanisms would "cure" the illness, if only given a chance to use its maximum vital force. Providing a "nudge" to the body's intelligence by giving small doses of a remedy that imitated the illness would invoke the natural action of the vital force.

The idea that, if kept in harmony, the body will be well is the key concept in chiropractic, as well as twentieth-century bodywork therapies, Rolfing, and Aston Patterning. In these fields of holistic health, most of the basic therapeutic techniques such as dietary change, herbal medicine, and physical manipulation are ancient Hippocratic approaches.

The diagnostic techniques in these traditions will by now seem familiar. Examining one part of the body to determine the whole, and asking questions about lifestyle are consistent throughout the great medical traditions of the Old World. In modern holistic health practices, this approach embraces iridology, reflexology, physiognomy and personology, the exhaustive symptoms lists of homeopathy, and body reading techniques in general. The latter consists of visually examining, touching, and manipulating the body to find areas of acute and chronic tension, pain, and "energy blockage."

Iridology and reflexology involve finding areas of "genetic" weakness, potential problem spots, by noticing features of the iris of the eye in iridology (Jensen 1952), in the hands and feet, and ultimately anywhere on the body in reflexology. Since each body part is a microcosm, a miniature hologram, of the larger being, any anatomical feature contains an energetic roadmap for the entire body (Molgaard 1979: 78–80). Iridology, used primarily to examine by proxy the state of the colon and circulation, mirrors the body's weaknesses by mapping the lesions, spots, rings, and colors of different parts of the iris. Each location corresponds to a part of the body. White, or perhaps brown wisps or clouds may appear at the apex of the iris. If the lines run from the area linked to the stomach to the head, this is considered evidence for a tendency for headaches, resulting in over-activity of the stomach (Kriege 1980: 72). Some configurations are temporary and reflect impermanent states. Concentric rings around the pupil, out to the edge of the iris, are called "nerve rings" and refer to the chronic emotional stress of the client. Similarly, a dark, but not black, scurf rim, encircling the iris refers to poor elimination. This is also a condition in flux. Practiced more often in Germany, its area of origin, iridology is solely a diagnostic, almost prognostic, technique. It does not provide a remedy. Herbs, cleansing diets, and exercise are the usual results of an iridology diagnosis.

Physiognomy—the practice of determining characteristics from physical features—is another Hippocratic diagnostic technique that infers the whole from the particular. The modern representative, personology, is primarily psychological, but it has implications for physical well-being. Mind and body are not separate. Like iridology, it is not designed to diagnose complicated acute conditions but to indicate general tendencies and potential threats to health. For example, the characteristic "tolerance" refers to the individual's emotional reaction to time. People who react impatiently, because they perceive time flowing quickly, possess "low tolerance." In personology, this trait is indicated by narrow spacing between the eyes. If the space between the eyes is narrower than the width of the eye, that means the person has a "low tolerance" (Whiteside n.d.: 45–46). Unlike iridology, a therapy is implicit in this procedure. A full diagnostic picture is intended to awaken "self-awareness" and individuals are taught to cope with their own once mysterious reactions. For the holistic health practitioner, this technique is meant to help him/her judge the client's reactions and recognize signs of stress. Practitioners are taught to notice the chronic stress lines that form and recognize where to look for tension and pain.

Asking questions is permitted in the diagnostic procedures of holistic health. In fact, it is often exhaustive. Unlike the rationalist, cosmopolitan medical tradition, disease is not a separable phenomenon. Diseases do not exist in holistic health, only imbalanced individuals. This concept is vital. It means no factor is truly irrelevant to the process of illness, particularly if that illness is perceived as an elimination. Medical histories become life histories (Vithoulkas 1981: 63–65). In homeopathy, the detail is so great a client is asked to keep a journal of thoughts, behaviors, desires, and aversions to help the homeopath decide precisely which syndrome and remedy are in question. The preference for cold food, or shade, or irritation caused by the neighbor's stereo might prove to be the key diagnostic features which separate this kind of headache from its myriad cousins (Hastings 1981: 463). For example, headache associated with heavy limbs and eyelids, hammering at the base of the brain, lack of thirst, and aggravated by tobacco, sunshine, and effort indicate Gelsemium as the most appropriate homeopathic remedy. This type of headache is most likely to be located in the forehead, coming on most often at 10 A.M. and is eased by lying down. Yet, a splitting headache, that feels as if a nail was being driven into the skull and that comes on after eating or upon rising results from overindulgence and responds to *nux vomica* (Anderson 1979: 44–47). This detailed inquiry has earned the title of encyclopedic nosology.

Chiropractic and bodywork therapies may use the aforementioned diagnostic techniques, but they also rely on visual, tactile, and in the case of chiropractic, mechanical examination. The practitioner watches the clients' range of motion and posture, looking for areas of tension and pain (Wilk 1976: 46). This may be done as a separate action or as part of the therapeutic routine. For example, it is easy to watch the body on the table adjust to its "normal" position and feel areas of tension or pain during a massage/bodywork session. It is possible to tactilely sense purely mechanical features, such as tension or inhibition. It is also part of the diagnostic training to learn to sense "energetic" qualities. One useful practice in holistic health practitioner training is learning to nonvisually sense heat and cold or emptiness and fullness in the area just above the physical body. These subtle sensations give clues about the client, just as a cramped muscle or a postural deviation does.

Deducing energy and emotional and physical states is only the prelude to manipulating these states. The techniques practiced most frequently in the study are naturopathy, natural hygiene, massage and bodywork therapy, and homeopathy, already discussed.

Naturopathic medicine is widespread for a practice that does not officially exist in Paraiso. The Naturopathic Doctor, an "N.D.," is not a legal status in California, yet the practices of naturopathy are intertwined with many holistic health practices. The "drugless therapists" of the early twentieth century are living well under different names. The principles of naturopathic medicine are straightforward. Behavioral and environmental impurity leads to the impairment of vital energy flow.

Cleansing, balancing, and tonifying are the mechanisms of reestablishing the "dynamic balance." Cleansing techniques embrace herbal cleansing, drinking water and flushing the system, enemas, and high colonics. The latter is a more involved and intensive enema, aimed at cleansing areas of the colon not usually accessible (Kloss 1971: 144). Fasting and dietary cleansing are the most critical techniques, although their intensity means they should be used with caution. They are the most powerful forms of stimulating elimination. Carrot juice, wheatgrass juice, sprouts, and fruit juices form the core of the purification diet. Exercise, particularly the use of slant boards and small trampolines, is used to encourage the flow of "cleansing lymph." Of course, massage and intensive bodywork are powerful purification tools. Again, this is done by improving circulation and breaking up "frozen" areas of the body.

Balancing and tonification are extensions of the purification process. Diets are changed to minimize further "pollution" and balance body minerals. At the very minimum, sugar, coffee, salt, preservatives, and additives are eliminated (Fadiman 1981: 255–56). Red meat and fats are reduced, although many feel any meat is spiritually demeaning (Ballentine 1979: 121; Christopher 1979: 518–43; Kalson and Kalson: 1979: 22; Mattson 1982: 84) and far too high on the ecological trophic scale (Christopher 1979: 536). The traditional association with vitamins and "health nuts" falls under the tonification rubric. It is very difficult to become truly pure. The spiritual, mental, emotional, and physical state of the environment precludes this. Once the body is clean, however, it can be strengthened to resist the onslaught of western civilization.

To illustrate the concept of toxicity and cleansing, I will return to the imaginary headache. As you might suspect, the cause of a headache in naturopathic medicine is usually poor eating and elimination and nervous distress. The balancing technique would focus on herbal and dietary changes, although the details, as you will see, vary. For a toxic headache, valerian, peppermint, spearmint, black cohash tea, or a cleansing flush of hot water and lemon could be administered. Another remedy recommends angelica, balmony, black alder, elecampagne, gentian root, raspberry and strawberry leaves, rhubarb, wild cherry, and wormwood in a tea. A tincture of lobelia is also applied locally (Christopher 1979: 27). Yet another concoction includes lobelia, cayenne (a powerful purifier), chamomile, peppermint, valerian, scullcap, wood betony, red clover blossoms, linden flowers and chaparral, comfrey, and elecampagne, along with vitamins A, B complex, C, and calcium (Montagna 1979: 71, 338–40). Nervous headaches would be soothed by an herbal concoction of peppermint, spearmint, catnip, and red sage or by a hops tea (Kloss 1971: 478–79). Most of the herbs are meant to soothe digestion and to tranquilize and purify the system, especially the blood. Massage is pertinent to either case, to relax the patient and stimulate the elimination of "toxins."

Natural hygiene is an extension and simplification of naturopathy. Once one of the more obscure disciplines within holistic health, the popularity of Harvey and Marilyn Diamond's book *Fit for Life* (1985), along with corresponding videotapes, media appearances, and surrounding controversy, has catapulated natural hygiene into the American national consciousness. In this paradigm, there is only one disease, *toxaemia.* Diet is the source and cure for all ill health. It is felt that Americans cook too much of their food, bolt it, and poison themselves with protein. This causes poor elimination, due to a lack of high water-content foods, infrequent use of fruit, and improper "food combining." In this system, fruit should be eaten alone, "proteins" and "starches" should never be mixed (M. Diamond 1980: vii–viii, 44; Diamond 1985; Goodman 1979: 138–39). Any deviation from this pattern will increase the chances of digestional putrefaction and create the toxins implied in toxaemia. It is a system that takes the idea of purification to an extreme, and its advocates are among the most zealous in the holistic health community.

In homeopathy, this philosophy is refined yet further. Elimination and rebalance are the ultimate goals. Miasms and ancient karmic and behavioral errors are expressed as illness (Concon 1980: 53; Vithoulkas 1981: 34–36; Weir 1972: 37–47). In homeopathy, practitioners hope to reverse the pattern. There are definite layers of illness that must be peeled off from the center outward, from the top down, and in reverse order of appearance. The first miasm is the last to go (Concon 1980: 55; Vithoulkas 1981: 98). A cure is effected by using minute doses of homeopathic remedies, recommended by the homeopath. However, the discipline required to shed the miasm remains the client's responsibility (Vithoulkas 1981: 68). These remedies are now produced in a variety of ways. All try to obtain an "energy imprint" of the physical substance that produces a similar set of symptoms (Vithoulkas 1980: 105; 1981: 20, 156). The basis for the imprints can be herbs, minerals, or virtually any potentially toxic substance. However, they must be specific to that unique combination of symptoms. The ingestion of such a substance sets off an immune response of the elan vital (Coulter 1979: 309). Although similar to immunology, there are some crucial differences. A vaccine, besides being far too material, is simply too general, too non-specific, to be homeopathic. For example, smallpox vaccine is designed to be effective for all, and so cannot be tailored to the individual. Some homeopathic remedies are weak and are easy to use. Bach flower remedies for emotional balance are in this category (Weeks 1979: 123). Others are "high potency," physically faint (some are below the minimum molecular weight of the physical substance) but active at the spirit level. These are difficult to use, requiring many hours of detailed diagnosis. These can, however, lead to a constitutional remedy, a panacea for that unique individual. This is the purest goal of a homeopath.

This paradigm is not consistent with orthodox medicine, or even, occasionally with herbal, naturopathic formulations. Any attempt to suppress pain or disease is antithetical to homeopathy. A long-standing, yet current, dividing point in homeopathy is whether this approach will be "mixed" with other medical techniques (Grossinger 1980: 1964– 67). This question of "mixers" and "straights" plagues the other highly professional school of healing, chiropractic.

Although the concept of elimination is not extinct in chiropractic, the aim is normalization of the body through physical manipulation. When the body, especially the spine, is correctly aligned, the homeostatic "Natural Intelligence" of the body can function to its greatest potential (Bricklin 1976: 100; Cowie 1975: 149–50; Maykovich 1980: 307–10; Wilk 1976: 25–46).

In chiropractic, postural deviation is corrected by adjusting the vertebral spinous and transverse processes. Abnormalities of the locomotor system, especially spine and pelvis are subluxations (Breen 1979: 73–77). Active manipulation, exercise, and postural education are legitimate tools of the "straight" chiropractors. This includes, not only the "adjustment" of the vertebral processes, but also massage, range of motion and yogic exercises, and advice on proper postures in potentially traumatic work or play. In addition, some other orthodox medical techniques may be adapted by the "mixers." The use of the chiropractic status to practice a blend of drugless therapies is, however, more common.

In theory, chiropractic can be used to alleviate any condition of ill health. In practice, it focuses on headaches, physical trauma, and chronic pain (Wilk 1976: 32). Some chiropractors are extremely specialized in the kind of treatment practiced or in the anatomical area treated. Not all chiropractors claim affiliation with the holistic health movement, in spite of common origins and shared philosophies. Yet, epistemologically, Chiropractic is close to most bodywork and massage therapies.

In the Hippocratic tradition, physical massage and manipulation are second only to diet as a source of therapy (Kellogg 1929: 11). In this legacy of tactile therapy, there is an astounding amount of variation. Bodywork may be intense and often painful in energy releasing traditions similar to the Ayurvedic tomasic style. Massage may also be sensitive, sensual, and soothing; this tradition, akin to the satvik, is gentle and designed to work at the spiritual, energetic level, balancing rather than breaking old patterns.

Intense bodywork is designed to break up frozen patterns of energy and the physical tension involved in those blocks. This can be done primarily at the energy level, using little visible effort, but acting in the "spirit plane." It can also be brought about by strong physical effort, clearly visible, and often initially agonizing. There are also techniques designed to tap into both systems. The complete gamut of bodywork therapies is practiced in Paraiso. In order of increasing materiality and intensity, these include:

> Attunement and Aura/energy balancing
> Finger-tapping/energy balancing
> Jin Shin Do
> Polarity-satvik
> Trager
> Orthobionomy
> Esalen and Swedish massage
> Swedish massage
> Shiatsu
> Polarity-tomasic
> Zone therapy/Reflex massage
> Deep tissue work (Rolfing etc.)

Practitioners often blend the therapies, depending on the needs and desire of the client. Bodywork oriented to light energy manipulation tends to be gentle and relaxing. This requires great concentration by the practitioner, for this work borders on psychic healing and involves careful visualization and "grounding." Satvik therapies work gently on the physical body and are intended to effect change by balancing the etheric aspects of a client. Constant attention must be paid to detecting subtle energy (coolness, heat, tingling, and pulse). Nurturing and painless, satvik therapies are passively received by the client. Priority is given to influencing energy. The training of a practitioner of orthobionomy illustrates this. The tools used are painless postural alignments, gentle rocking, light touching, or "off-the-body" balancing. Initially the focus is on anatomical postural positioning. A tense limb is placed in such a way that pain is relieved and the client is asked about whether pain is felt. A more advanced technique requires increased sensitivity. The client is no longer asked, the practitioner can "feel" the release. The most advanced forms bypass physical sensation and focus on balancing the aura, literally divining the source of imbalance. Adjustment takes place a few inches from the physical body. Empathy is all important.

The degree to which the practitioner seeks empathy differs. For example, in orthobionomy, the client's energy is "good." Love and light unite the client and practitioner. Energetic contact is not something to guard against or avoid. For disciplines other than orthobionomy, making sure that the empathy is not overdone is a priority. Excessive empathy in this kind of bodywork is believed by some to endanger the practitioner, bringing the client's ills to the therapist. In this work, the practitioner is a conduit, not a source, of healing elan vital.

Midrange massage therapies, such as Esalen, Swedish, and shiatsu massage are clearly physical, sometimes soothing, occasionally intense (Frager 1981: 216–20). They act primarily on the physical body, although shiatsu is based on the acupuncture meridians. These are the most common and popular brands of bodywork.

Tomasic therapies, Polarity, reflex massage, and deep tissue manipulation, like Rolfing, are intended to radically alter the energy/physical configuration of the body (Gilchrist 1972: 4–10). This usually means actively pressing, kneading, hacking, or twisting the body in such a way that old patterns are traumatically realigned. From the point of view of the practitioner and the client, it is easily the most dramatic agent of change. Amidst the screams and flailing limbs, it becomes easy to believe that something is happening.

Like chiropractic, in theory, bodywork can be used to alleviate any acute or chronic condition. It aids elimination, it directly or indirectly affects energy, it relaxes and lets the body's native intelligence rebalance. Practitioners are most clearly taught, however, about chronic conditions, overall tonification, and corporeal education. Pain, chronic tension, and postural deviation have become the ad hoc realm of bodywork.

Within this framework, specific syndromes such as headaches or backaches can be affected. Some therapies, such as reflexology or zone therapy specifically address such a problem. In zone therapy, each body part reflects another. The thumb and big toe "reflect" the head. The web between thumb and first digit is a reflex of the neck and shoulders. Concentrating pressure on these areas is meant to directly relieve a headache (Carter 1980a: 97–100; 1980b: 37–38). Naturally, in massage in general, a headache could also be influenced by direct kneading, hacking, chucking, tapping, flexing or, stroking of the neck, shoulders, and head (Kellogg 1929: 119; 278–79). Moreover, a less physical approach can also be used. Placing hands on either side of the face, with fingers touching points along the face, is a satvik technique, relaxing the client and restoring energetic balance.

HEALING WITH MIND AND SPIRIT

In holistic health the psyche clearly refers to both mind and soul. Rarely does a "holistic" psychotherapy direct itself to the mind and emotions without also addressing a spiritual or religious issue. The doctrines may have been partially reworked through scientific terminology, but orgone energy, "visualization and imagination therapy" still refer to elan vital and meditation. Archetypes and the collective unconscious are used as if they refer to nearly magical, mystical devices. They intertwine, and this intersection should be acknowledged. Yet despite an overlap, the psychological and psychic holistic health therapies are distinct enough to be considered separately.

There is a range of activities sometimes called "innovative psychotherapies." As we shall see in chapter 5, they developed in several leaps in the 1930s and 1960s. Wilhelm Reich, Carl Jung, Fritz Perls, Abraham Maslow, and a host of less well-known theoreticians led the way in reinstituting humanism and metaphysics in psychology. Reich's orgone therapy and Perls' Gestalt have had the heaviest impact on the creation of holistic health psychotherapies. Reich's followers, Charles Kelly and Alexander Lowen, created the active branches of Neo-Reichian therapy, Radix, and Bioenergetics. Flowing from Esalen, California, the Mecca of holistic health, Gestalt has been incorporated in Polarity and in sensitivity training sessions and has fed back into Neo-Reichian work.

Releasing suppressed traumas and creating new and purer patterns is inherent in the belief system of innovative psychologies. Emotion reflects higher energies. In Reichian therapy, breath is the key to orgone energy, just as it is the source of ch'i and prana. Releasing developmental (if not karmic) muscular holding patterns, known as armour, is the goal. The source of that armouring is coloured by sexuality (Grossinger 1980: 274–76). The variations in accomplishing this aim are enormous. Some therapists, the "Paleo-Reichians," prefer to work solely with sound, the breath, and gentle touching to slowly get the muscular armouring to unfold (Baker 1981: 599–603). Neo-Reichian therapy can be much more dramatic and overtly sexual, and the associated bodywork might well be more intense and physically active.

Gestalt therapy is used with bodywork and releasing postures in Polarity therapy and in group sessions. In practice, it locates the areas of karmic difficulty, one's "work." Role playing, particularly with phantom parents, siblings and spouses, and occasionally therapists, brings up a karmic lesson (see Perls 1969: 18, 60, 252). The spiritual burden may be anger at being born female, hatred of filial duty, or inability to take the therapist at his word. Roles are played out under the supervision of a therapist. He/she is trained to pick out key words, such as "I'll try" or "yes, but" and to immediately point out the attempt by the client to avoid the critical issue. Particularly emotive phrases are repeated by the client until emotions flow freely, and the initial attitude is changed. This is the affective aspect of the concept of elimination.

Just as postures are used in t'ai chi ch'uan and yoga to encourage spiritual and energetic change, movement and postural therapy facilitates emotional reflection and self-awareness (Green 1981: 95–96). Aston Patterning, dance therapy, and techniques of Alexander (Carrington 1972) and Feldenkreis (1972) use imagery, self-inspection, and movement reeducation to "realign the spirit." For example, in Aston Patterning, a client's walk could be examined, perhaps by watching imprints on a beach. The practitioner may observe that the feet are being strained to rotate inward, with the soles of the feet leaning toward the medial line. Pelvic tension may be the culprit. Bodywork, imagery, and range of motion movements could be used to free the block. Visualization can be employed using white light to "thaw" the block, or to explore the basic fear behind the pelvic armouring (see Halprin and Khalighi 1982: 79; Mattson 1982: 180). Visualization may take on a religious content. For example, in dance therapy, one can "dance" the emotions of suffering and humiliation until the emotion and the movement fill the client's mind. Specific religious imagery of a compassionate Buddha is invoked. The client is meant to be filled with forgiveness. Then the therapist "guides" the image of the Buddha away, to be replaced by the client's image. Every person contains the Buddha, so self-forgiveness is possible. This is an explicitly spiritual exercise.

There is an area of innovative psychology, christened stress reduction, that is essential in the lifestyles of holistic health practitioners and clientele (Mattson 1982: 28). Meditation, hypnosis, self-hypnosis, and visualization are the primary techniques in this mode (Samuels 1980; Schulz 1981: 383–87; Shames and Sterin 1978; Shorr 1981: 684–98). These therapies often border on the mystical. Buddhist *Zazen,* Transcendental Meditation (T.M.), breathing meditations, Rosicrucian mystical rose meditations, and guided visualizations are relaxation techniques. Visualization sometimes gives clues to cognitive and emotional problems (Hastings 1981: 466). Such techniques are also theurgic devices, designed through ritual activity to elevate the nature of the soul. Moreover, cheerfully chatting with spirit guides (see Mattson 1982: 17) and archetypes in a state of self-hypnosis is clearly an attempt to achieve an altered state of consciousness. It can be used to gain power as a potential practitioner, as well as knowledge. In one exercise, a client or novice practitioner is guided into a safe place in the nether regions of his/her mind. There, the client is introduced to "the child." The child is the client, at age five, in the most abstract form. The child becomes a guardian spirit, helping to reinstitute a spirit of fun and play. In turn, the adult client takes responsibility for "the child." They exchange gifts and become friends. These imaginary forays into the world of archetypes are a way of manipulating energy. This kind of innovative psychology links the physical/emotional therapies in holistic health to the esoteric.

Psychic healing in holistic health practice is expressed as a component of other practices (Mattson 1982: 17). It is also a separate skill/calling. Being able to directly "sense" etheric energy is a useful diagnostic talent in a system where energy is the basis of all illness and therapy. If in no other way, the assumptions of reincarnation, karma, spiritual realms, and spiritual evolution are pervasive. Practitioners, constantly exposed to other people's often unhealthy "energies," want to find a way to protect themselves. The more effective a practitioner's skill in moving energy, the greater the danger of stirring up a psychic force or entity that cannot be handled. "Grounding," making sure that the energy does not flow from the client to the healer, and making sure that energy flows without draining the practitioner are considered *psionic* skills. They are derived from the occult arts. The last thing a practitioner wants is to attract "negative energy," which can make him/her imbalanced and ill.

Basic protective skills start with acquiring sensitivity to the body's "subtle energy," the aura, and stretching the imagination to the point where visualizations can be made manifest at will. "Seeing" auras, being able to visualize astral havens, and directing an ideal energy stream are the fundamentals. Being able to question archetypes and establish relationships with spirit guides are more advanced, but essential psychic skills. Spirit guides are a widely held Spiritualist belief. Each individual has at least two, male and female. They are aspects of one's own self, guardians on the higher planes. The guides can advise, warn, answer questions, and eventually aid in diagnoses. However, the guides do whatever is best for their charge's karma. This may mean pain and suffering, if that is what is necessary to improve the spirit. The guides cannot be used as genies, particularly by psychic novices. Most of the holistic healers I observed did not pursue psychic healing as the main avenue of therapy. It is an approach used as a secondary tool while the practitioner used other techniques involving bodywork or counseling. In a session, the practitioner may even use visualization without the client's awareness.

Psychic healers, unlike most practitioners of holistic health, practice from a talent or calling rather than as a learned skill. Their keen perception of the esoteric and their commitment to "higher" realms gives them status in the community. There are only a handful of psychic healers in Paraiso, and competition is somewhat fierce. Healers promote the status of their guides and their ability to function in the spirit realm. Sensing auras or aspects of the client's soul are the diagnostic keys. For example, karmic strings may be visualized around the heads of practitioners who do not ground themselves properly. Color and intensity of the aura and the Indian or Tibetan chakras indicate the spiritual basis of emotional or physical problems. These problems can be directly affected through the innate healing power of the individual or by the healer's power to channel higher forms of energy. Therapy relies on a complex system of causation. However, the assumptions of healers are historically wrapped up in the philosophical antecedents of holistic health. The imagery of psychic healing and the esoteric colors the millennial and revitalistic visions of the future within the wider holistic health community.

The various techniques used by holistic health workers are the products of geographically diverse origins and creative syntheses, linked by common symbolic concerns. Like other social movements holistic health is brought together by both symbols and networking. By understanding the assumptions, causative models, diagnostic and therapeutic practices used we can extract elements of the symbolic system behind them. The cosmological assumptions, the perceptions of causation, create a certain way of looking at things. The focus on purity, elimination, and an overwhelming sense of responsibility color the holistic health movement. Even before the dawn of Aquarian consciousness in the 1960s, the techniques and assumptions existed. Chapter 4 documents the historical processes antecedent to holistic health.

THE ROOTS OF HOLISTIC HEALTH

For I am the wisdom of the Greeks and the knowledge of the barbarians. (from the Gnostic text, "The Thunder, Perfect Mind" [Barnstone 1984: 596])

The belief systems of modern holistic health stem from ancient conceptions that were long established in the Hippocratic, Ayurvedic, and East Asian medical traditions. The principles that are fundamental to the holistic health movement existed long before 1960. They include the introduction of the following practices and beliefs: 1) the separable soul, forerunner of "vital essence," 2) elements as impersonal forces in nature, 3) dietary therapy, 4) the colon as the root of disease, 5) diagnosis of the whole from the part (for example, pulse diagnosis), 6) healing crises and elimination, 7) the nature of causation and the role of uncertainty in medicine, 8) the role of physician as practitioner or philosopher (scientist), 9) naturalism, 10) self-responsibility, and 11) the role of karma and reincarnation.

The three traditions blended and interacted in the formation of holistic health. It is crucial to realize that these systems have also interacted in the past. They were not isolated, closed structures of knowledge, huddling in various corners of the Old World. The exchange of assumptions and materia medica created a greater system of naturalistic medicine that lent itself to repeated syntheses.

This historical process has important implications for today's holistic health practitioners because it provides a formal historical position, a justification for regularizing the liminal status of an alternative healer. The need for a legitimizing tradition is recognized by the legal defenders of the field (Green 1978a: 390). If holistic health practitioners are perceived by others as upstart synthesists of various imports and archaic superstitions, they cannot establish a firm place within the larger society. Holistic healers neither embrace established religion nor practice orthodox medicine, two legally recognized healing traditions.

Holistic health practitioners must find a way to legitimize their practices with established authority, while rebelling against it. They lack the option of relying on the authority of their current founding mothers and fathers. No court is going to respond to the insights of Wilhelm Reich or the incorporation of bits and pieces of imported Indian and Chinese practices. The weight of historical tradition, however, is an authority that is more difficult to refute. Acknowledging ancient roots is a possible strategy of institutionalization.

The discovery of the depth behind the tradition of holistic health also stimulates some anthropological inquiry. The antecedents of a social movement are part of an open, not closed, system. Historical research cannot legitimately focus only on Carl Jung's Switzerland, Daniel Palmer's midwestern America, or Fritz Perls's California, but must look further back. Reciprocal diffusion of medicine and religious philosophy in the Old World was widespread. These traditions are all based on a similar system of physics and on major compilations stemming from ancient oral traditions, codified within centuries of one another. The mysterious similarities between the three major historical traditions become less opaque when the periodic interchange of ideas and practices is revealed.

The survival of ancient traditions has implications for the overall process of a social movement. The notion of inevitable, premature death for non-institutionalized social movements becomes less believable when looking at a 2500 year old tradition.

The holistic health movement was born of a mixture of orthodox and heretical traditions. Some periods of the traditions' development did involve institutionalization. What could be more hierarchical and routinized than imperial Chinese medicine? At the same time, much of the epistemology and practice of empirical medicine in Europe was part of a sub-rosa tradition. How did it survive? Robert Ellwood suggests a parallel process to the transfer of knowledge in a shamanistic tradition. Each individual seeks his own unique worldview but within known cultural parameters (1973: 8–22). It is important not to confuse the lack of a visible social structure with a cultural void. Informal, decentralized structures also pass on critical cultural information. No anthropologist, studying a social movement, should lose sight of this.

The act of compiling historical information provided anthropological insights. It reinforced my understanding of the integration of culture. I did not get a clear picture of the history of empirical medicine, by looking at the historiography of only political/economic events, or religion/philosophy, or even medicine. Examining history holistically—meshing political, religious, and medical spheres—produced a thought-provoking historical image.

Even the biases of historians provided clues to the evolution of alternative medicine. Themes of nationalism and the quest for spiritual truths pervaded the pages of the history of medicine and religion. Once again, the desire to legitimize social identity through history influenced the historians' interpretation of events and dates. Classicists desiring antiquity pushed back the dates of Greek medicine and philosophy. Indian historians also sought ancient dates, and the others found a way for the Chinese to be the founding fathers of all medicine and religion. Historical "apologists" for various cultures and religious affiliations promoted different versions of religious, medical, and political history. I have tried to reconcile the various scenarios, through my own biases, and produce the chronology presented in this chapter.

The holistic health movement, and perhaps almost any movement, does not spring forth fully grown. This is an illusion. Visible jumps in history are preceeded by a long series of mundane events and perhaps by other hierarchical leaps. These leaps may not be immediately evident. The production of each of the major ideas in holistic health, listed at the beginning of this chapter, was a significant leap. Viewed together, they produce a continuous tradition. General histories, or even histories of medicine and philosophy are designed to describe the chain of events leading to orthodox medical science not to holistic health. Ambitiously, this chapter is constructed to illuminate the background of the holistic health movement that has appeared in the last 150 years.

NOT FROM THE HEAD OF ZEUS

Using literature in patristics (the study of early Christianity), medieval, medical, religious, scientific, and esoteric history as well as some primary sources in naturalistic medicine and the occult, I pieced together a chronology of events and ideas that relate to modern holistic health in Paraiso. The emphasis is on European history, for the movement was born in Europe and her cultural colonies.

Three categories of events emerged. These three domains—political, philosophical and medical history—are presented comparatively in the columns of the chronology of the development of empirical medicine in India, China, Europe, and finally America and Paraiso in Figures 4.1 through 4.8. The chronology is divided into historical periods of exchange. In one era, the Persians might have been the culture brokers, in the next the Hellenists, followed by Romans and Christians, Arabs, Persians, and European colonials. Each produced a period of eclecticism and reciprocal exchange. Political and economic exchange through warfare, trade, and religious evangelism linked populations throughout the Old World. Exchanges created networks for the trade of information. The political stability brought about by geographic integration in the Persian Achaemenian, Alexandrian, Ptolemaic, Seleucid, Roman, Indian Mauryan, and Chinese Han empires further facilitated exchange. The expansion of Islam and European colonialism are examples of political history's impact on information exchange. Trade in spices and drugs, mercenaries and missionaries were also part of this continuing process.

Ideas about the nature of man and causation often filtered through religious and philosophical interchange. These ideas were foreign to the cultures that enthusiastically embraced the new beliefs. For example, the Greek philosophical interpretation of foreign ecstatic shamanic states produced Pythagoreans, Gnostics, Neoplatonists, hermeticists, and eventually Christian heretics. All used an "alien" concept to pursue a course of mysticism. The content and thrust was synthetic, blending influences from Thracian shaman to Brahmanic philosophers. This tradition was continued in the esoteric beliefs of medieval European magi and mystical (and often heretical) movements in Islam and Christianity. Swedenborg, Mesmer, Freemasons, and transcendentalists continued this pursuit. The explosion of Spiritualism, New Thought, and Theosophy created networks ripe for holistic health.

Ancient naturalistic medical systems evolved through time, often exchanging metaphysical and physical ideas and the material tools of the craft. Ayurvedic, Chinese, and advocates of Hippocratic systems were periodically interlocked. From the fifth century B.C. to the second century of the Christian Era, Hippocratic medicine debated the epistemological basis for the empirical medical system, the parent of holistic health, and the rationalistic medical system, now dubbed "Western" medicine. The two systems have existed side by side since the second century.

THE LINKS ARE FORGED

It is easy to forget that the development of naturalistic medicine in the early urban environment was not isolated to either the Indus Valley in India, or the Yellow River in China, or to the island of Cos, birthplace of Hippocrates. The movements of migrants, merchants, pilgrims, and armies cut wide swaths throughout Asia and the Mediterranean world. Much of the historical literature attempts to find the "origin" of a given trait or idea and to document its diffusion. Occasionally, scholars will take the approach that the diffusion was reciprocal. Ideas, observations, and packets of herbs were easy to exchange. The result was not a pure stream of Indian, Egyptian, Mesopotamian, Chinese, or Greek thought that poured from its source but rather bastardized adoptions of imported ideas, following pre-existing networks of trade, conquest, and migration. My analytical task was to identify the networks and document philosophical and medical exchanges.

The naturalistic medical systems themselves formed along pre-existing networks. Long before the codification of Indian or Greek thought, prior connections had developed in the Harappan-Bahrein-Mesopotamian sea routes and Persian and Afghani overland routes during the period of 2500 to 1700 B.C. (Asthana 1976: 37–51; Filliozat 1964: 34; Thorwald 1962: 182). Map 4.1 illustrates these exchange patterns.

These connections created lines of communication that were repeatedly reinforced. The Indo-Iranian connection of the sixth century B.C. is clearly related to the development of naturalistic medicine (Filliozat 1964: 37). By this time the idea of wind as a life force was

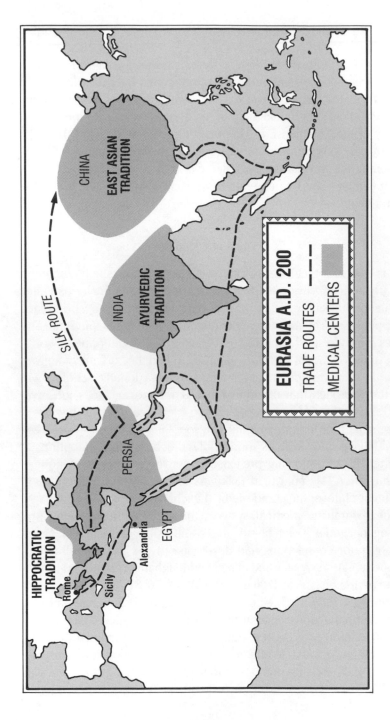

MAP 4.1   NATURALISTIC MEDICAL CENTERS OF THE OLD WORLD

clearly developed in both Vedic and Iranian thought. This was the forerunner of elemental and vitalistic concepts in modern holistic health.

In seventh century B.C. India, The Lokayata school of thought debated the metaphysics of the elements. Are there five, including earth, air, fire, water and the intangible *akasha,* ether? The Lokayata school dropped the ether, and their materialist physics reciprocally influenced both Greek and Chinese medicine (Mahdihassan 1979: 316; Huard and Wong 1968: 91), although they lost the debate in some schools of Ayurvedic medicine.

In Europe, the early Apollonian Greeks were exposed to ecstatic shamanism in Thrace and Scythia. The stage was set for speculation about out-of-body phenomena, the separation of the soul and the pursuit of immortality (Dodds 1951: 140; Ellwood 1973: 43–47). By the seventh century B.C. the trade contacts had become colonies, and spiritualist ideas flourished in Orphism (see Figure 4.1). In the sixth century B.C. the dominant political force was the Achaemenian empire of Persia that existed until Alexander. It created stability from India to Greece and even supported an Indian merchant colony in Memphis, Egypt, from 525–405 B.C. (Asthana 1976: 170; Filliozat 1964: 239–44; Upadhyaya 1973: 58), and perhaps through the Ptolemaic reign (Prakash 1964: 249). In this era Buddhism began, and the philosopher Pythagoras drew on Greek shamanism/ Orphism and his experiences in India to create his own school of thought (Dodds 1951: 144–45; Ellwood 1973: 50–52). The ideas of Pythagoras—the separation and perfection of the soul over matter, asceticism, and the pursuit of immortality—left a stamp on European esoteric thought (Coulter 1975: 103). Books containing these concepts are still found in metaphysical bookshelves in Paraiso. The Theosophical Institute in Camino Robles is even named after his school, Krotona.

In Egypt, priests found that putrification began in the colons of mummies. This discovery led to theories on the origin of diseases. Greek mercenaries brought these Egyptian medical ideas back to be incorporated later into the Cnidian School of Hippocratic medicine (Saunders 1963: 7–15). This contact paved the way for the naturopathic concept of the colon as the source point for disease.

Even China was not isolated, but absorbed Babylonian astrological ideas into its sixfold categories of yin and yang (see Figure 3.1) in the sixth century B.C. (Needham and Gwei-Djen 1969: 259). Without such categories, pulse diagnosis and acupuncture would be quite different.

FIGURE 4.1 A CHRONOLOGY OF THE EMPIRICAL MEDICAL TRADITION:
700–400 B.C., THE CREATION OF THE TRADITIONS

POLITICAL/ ECONOMIC HISTORY	PHILOSOPHICAL HISTORY	MEDICAL HISTORY
SEVENTH CENTURY B.C.		
Europe: Greek Colonies in Thrace, Scythia Egypt: 663–609 B.C. Introduction of Greek Mercenaries	India: Lokayata materialist drop akasha, leaves four elements	
SIXTH CENTURY B.C.		
Europe; Asia; Persia; India: 525–331 B.C. Achaemenian Persian Empire Egypt: 525–405 B.C. Indian merchant colony in Memphis, under Persian domination	Europe: Orphism—Immortality and separation of the soul; Pythagoras (580 to 500 B.C.), philosopher, travels to India, founds Krotona in Italy India: Buddhism is founded	China: Influence of Babylonian State Astrology on sixfold yin/yang classification; creation of pharma- ceutical texts
FIFTH CENTURY B.C.		
		Europe: Creation of Sicilian School of medicine, (physicians as philosophers) influenced Plato

Professionalization in naturalistic medicine had begun. In China, the medical system was not yet developed, but standardized pharmaceutical texts were already being produced (Unschuld 1977a: 112). Only a century later, debates had begun in Greece. Did the physician practice a professional craft, or was he a special kind of philosopher? The Sicilian school promoted the latter belief, influencing Plato and later Aristotle and foreshadowing the rationalist/empiricist debate (Coulter 1975: 117).

The fourth century B.C. was a turning point for naturalistic medicine. The Achaemenian empire collapsed, to be replaced by Alexander's Hellenistic hegemony, including the Ptolemaic dynasty in Egypt and the Seleucids in west Asia (see Figure 4.2). Taking no chances, Alexander supported an eclectic range of physicians, including the use of Indian expertise in snakebites and Indian epidemic disease (Asthana 1976: 204). His mentor, Aristotle (384–322 B.C.) gained a prominence that was reflected in the Aristotelean rationalist school. Rationalists held that causes were knowable, and knowing the cause, solutions were possible. This concept, as you will soon see became a matter of hot debate in Hippocratic medicine. The Sceptics of the third century B.C. denied the ability to know cause from materialist deduction and preceeded the formation of the empirical school of thought (Coulter 1975: 173).

Hippocratic physicians in the fourth century B.C. continued to struggle with the nature of disease etiology. The Cnidian school favored the Egyptian concept that disease started with intestinal putrefaction (Coulter 1975: 110; Saunders 1963: 21–22). Cos, the school of Hippocrates, leaned toward an explanation of disease based on humoral pathology. For example, an excess of fire would be treated by reducing the heat, through dietary changes, herbs, and manipulations. This idea developed reciprocally with Indian thought. During this period, the Hippocratic Corpus was compiled from the works of both Coan and Cnidian schools (Lloyd 1978: 9–10).

The standardization of the naturalistic traditions continued. In India, the *Charaka Samhita,* an Ayurvedic commentary (based on an oral tradition) was compiled. The dates vary widely on this document from 600 B.C. (Dube 1978: 209) to A.D. 100 (Basham 1977: 20–21; Dunn 1976: 149). The *Susruta Samhita,* the second major commentary on Ayurvedic medicine, was created between 800 B.C. and A.D. 400 (Dube 1978: 209; Thorwald 1962: 202), although probably after the *Charaka Samhita* was written.

From the fourth century B.C. to the beginning of the Christian Era, the centers of medicine—India, Persia, China, and the Hellenistic world—were creatively interactive. From 297 B.C. to 150 A.D., the Mauryan dynasty stabilized large sections of India. The Mauryan kings sent medical supplies and expertise to the Seleucid Hellenists, and fostered a period of philosphical and medical exchange (Upadhyaya 1973: 45–48). During the second century B.C., Buddhist missionaries began

FIGURE 4.2 A CHRONOLOGY OF THE EMPIRICAL MEDICAL TRADITION: 399–100 B.C., THE HELLENISTIC SYNTHESIS

POLITICAL/ ECONOMIC HISTORY	PHILOSOPHICAL HISTORY	MEDICAL HISTORY
FOURTH CENTURY B.C.		
Europe to India: Alexander the Great (356–323 B.C.) Uses Indian Physicians for Indian diseases	Europe: Aristotle (384–322 B.C.) Founder of Rationalist School	Europe: Egyptian concept of putrefaction is exported to Cnidos (407–357 B.C.); Hippocratic Corpus compiled (430–330 B.C.), combining Greek Coan and Cnidian schools
Egypt: 323–30 B.C. Ptolemaic dynasty		
Asia Minor: 312–64 B.C. Seleucid Dynasty		
		China: Uses Babylonian mercurial preparations; also obtains five element concept from India
THIRD CENTURY B.C.		
India: 297 B.C.–A.D. 150 Mauryan Empire— Mauryan kings present Seleucids with Indian materia medica, reciprocal exchange with Asian Greeks	Europe: Skeptics—forerunners of Empiricist thought in medicine	China: *Huang-Ti nei Ching* is compiled 300 B.C.–A.D. 1st century range, (commentaries A.D. 700)
SECOND CENTURY B.C.		
Europe: 190 B.C. Rome begins gaining control of the Hellenized world		Europe/Africa: Buddhist missionaries bring Indian medicine to Hellenistic Syria
Persia, India: 100 B.C. Silk routes to China begin		China: Second century B.C. Pulse diagnosis taken to Tibet, then India, Arab/Persian world and finally to Europe by A.D. 1700
China: 200 B.C.– A.D. 200 Han dynasties stabilize trade routes		

to travel to the Hellenized Middle East (Bashram 1977: 22; Needham 1970: 40), bringing salvation and medical practices.

During this period, the Chinese were adding fundamental aspects to their medical repertoire. In the fourth century B.C. the Chinese began to use Babylonian mercurial preparations in the pursuit of longevity. Elemental concepts, borrowed from India, formed the outline of the five elemental phases (Agren 1975; Huard and Wong 1968: 12–16). These five, along with the sixfold yin/yang conception form the basis for meridians and for theoretical Chinese medicine. Once this had been accomplished the oral tradition was compiled in such classics as the *Yellow Emperor's Classic of Internal Medicine,* the *Huang-ti nei Ching* (see Vieth 1972), in the third century B.C. (Porkert 1976; 70; Vieth 1972: 7; Wang 1979: 295), although some scholars place it at a later time (Foster and Anderson 1978: 62; Needham and Gwei-Djen 1969: 262)

By 190 B.C. two political events had an impact on the potential for exchange for the next four centuries. These were the rise of the Roman empire in the Mediterranean and the Han dynasty in China. Overland and sea routes had become considerably more stable, and the silk route began by 100 B.C. (Barraclough 1982: 24). Greco-Egyptian, Syrian, and Lebanese traders, under the auspices of the Roman Empire, opened sea ports in India until the third century of the Christian Era (Needham 1970: 41). The exchange of goods was accompanied by an exchange of medical knowledge. The expertise of Chinese pulse diagnosis made its way to Tibet, then India, and centuries later into the Arab/Persian sphere, only arriving in Europe in the 1600s (Huard in Needham and Gwei-Djen 1969: 291).

THE EMPIRICIST/RATIONALIST DEBATE

A critical issue in the formation of the Hippocratic medical tradition was the debate between the empiricists and the rationalists. This schism is far more important for the history of holistic health than the medical historical split between the schools of Cos and Cnidos over the etiology of disease in elemental imbalance or digestive putrefaction. The epistemological split endured and eventually produced the holistic health and orthodox medical positions. The split revolved around the role of the healer and the qualities of nature—human and physical.

In the fifth century B.C., the Sicilian school began to promote the idea of physician as philosopher. The question ran, is a physician primarily a craftsman whose goal is healing, or a philosopher/scientist who seeks knowledge? This is a watershed decision. If the physician is a craftsman, then he studies the empirical results of remedies and does not concern himself with the workings of the cosmos. The only valuable area of research is the empirical tabulation of observations after the treatment is administered. Deduction can play no part where causes are not knowable. Indeed, the empirical practitioner may believe that knowledge of true cause and effect is not even possible, let alone fruitful. Causes are inseparable from each other and the patient. There are no diseases, only diseased persons. Moreover, the highest force in the universe is spirit, not available to the workings of the rational human mind.

It was the task of the empirical physician to thoroughly understand the characteristics of that particular individual patient, and know a "remedy" that would engage the natural homeostatic mechanisms of the individual. The remedies varied over the centuries from the regimens of exercise and diet. The use of provocative herbs aided *pepsis,* the burning of impurities, inducing a "healing crisis" while the body cured itself. The latest expression of this was in homeopathy and naturopathy, both designed to invoke the body's defenses and "eliminate" the miasm or toxins through a healing crisis (Coulter 1975; 11, 484–507).

For the scientist/philosopher, on the other hand, cure follows the definition of cause. Causes are isolatable and knowable. For the rationalist, seeking cause is the single most valuable area of inquiry. Once a cause is known, a rational deduction can be made about treatment, by balancing humors, if that is the prevailing paradigm (Levine 1971: 255), or injecting an antibiotic in a later understanding of nature. Etiology is not based on correspondence or kinship of the variables, but linear cause and effect (Foucault 1973: 11). Rationalist medicine is primarily a materialistic system and spiritual factors are not vital. Individual causes are separable and adjunct variables can be controlled. The fruition of this approach in the nineteenth century conceptually separated the disease entity from the human carrier (Coulter 1975: 16; Foucault 1973: 14; Treacher and Wright 1982: 3–4). Philosopher/scientists could look at leprosy, sans the leper. This is a uniquely rationalist position, and it is conceptually impossible in the empiricist approach. The two are fundamentally different.

Although Chinese and Ayurvedic medicine can also be highly deductive and materialistic, there is an undercurrent of induction (Porkert 1976: 63), spirituality, and concern with psychology (Huard and Wong 1968: 34). Their integration and holism lend themselves to the empirical approach. Unschuld points out that even though the philosophy of empiricism was promoted by Samuel Hahnemann (creator of homeopathy), it could even more accurately be used to describe Chinese medicine (1973: 46, 47, 172, my translation). In Asian medicine, causes, even elemental ones, remain remarkably elusive and empiricism prevails in actual practice (American Herbal Pharmacology Delegation 1975: 4–12).

In summary, empiricists and rationalists perceive the nature of reality differently. Empirical knowledge is linked with individual experience, unique to each person. Absolute, orthodox knowledge that exists separately from individual perception is not the empirical mode. It is not surprising the empiricists were so readily incorporated into the mystical tradition in the second century of the Christian Era or that the rationalists became the schoolmen of orthodoxy.

HERESIES, SPIRITUAL AND MEDICAL

While the empiricist/rationalist debate was born in Greece, the formation of formal schools took place in the Roman Empire (see Figure 4.3). The onset of Christianity, and the influx of Hellenistic and oriental religious disciplines sharpened the epistemological distinctions. Gnostic and heretical Christians—as they were later defined by the orthodoxy—and Pythagorean Hellenistic philosophers, such as Apollonius of Tyana promoted the idea of a mystical, personal quest for truth, one that existed for the spirit, not the material illusion. This period of vision quests and heretical pronouncements went on through the third century.

Eclectic syntheses proliferated exponentially. Once truth relies on personal revelation, not on orthodox dogma, there are few boundaries to the number of truths possible. The Gnostics, and later the Theosophists, learned this lesson. Virtually each generation of disciples found

FIGURE 4.3 A CHRONOLOGY OF THE EMPIRICAL MEDICAL TRADITION:
A.D. 1–300, HERESIES, SPIRITUAL AND MEDICAL

POLITICAL/ ECONOMIC HISTORY	PHILOSOPHICAL HISTORY	MEDICAL HISTORY
FIRST CENTURY A.D.		
Europe: first to third Century Roman (i.e. Greco-Egyptian, Syrian, Lebanese) ports in India	Europe: Christianity founded 35 A.D.; Apollonius of Tyana, a Pythagorean, travels to India, founds a school that lasts until fifth century A.D.	India: *Charaka Samhita* is compiled in a range of 600 B.C.–A.D. 100; After this, the *Susruta Samhita* is written within a range from 800 B.C.–A.D. 400
SECOND CENTURY A.D.		
	Europe: A.D. 100–160 Marcion (90?–160) Christian theologian denies importance of Judaism; Valentinus (+100–160) Christian Gnostic, Hellenistic synthesist, taught in Rome A.D. 135–160	Europe: Galen (129–199), stabilizes Rationalist school of medicine; Celsus d. 185 formalized empirical school in Rome
	India: Christian missionaries sent to India second to fourth centuries	
THIRD CENTURY A.D.		
	Europe: Plotinus (205–270) founder of Neo-platonism, pagan Gnostic philosopher, hellenized Egyptian; later followed by theurgic Neoplatonists and hermeticists, including Iamblichus (250–325)	Europe: +200 Sextus Empiricus last official Empirical physician, empiricism enters the esoteric tradition until thirteenth century

a new path to follow. The critical points at issue were the relationship to Judaism, the nature of the local versus ultimate divinity, and the superiority of spirit over thought and matter. The inherent illusion of *hyle*, matter, logically led to the rejection of rationalist materialism.

Indian religious concepts, which by this point were almost indistinguishable from Pythagorean ideas, seeped into Christian and pagan thought (Prakash 1964: 253) and were bent in the process. In the first century, the pagan Apollonius had travelled to India while in the army. He returned to found a philosophical/mystical school. Christian missionaries were being sent to India by the second century (Upadhyaya 1973: 58). Even those on the borderline of orthodoxy, such as the theologian Origen, postulated the pre-existence of the soul, although he rejected transmigration as heresy (Dodds 1965: 128; G. R. S. Mead 1967: 84). Some Christian Gnostics embraced transmigration, a concept akin to Buddhist or Hindu rebirth, but found the entrapment in the inherently sinful hyle revolting and sought secret teaching to aid their escape (Barnstone 1984: 266–288: Pagels 1981; Walker 1983). Pagan Gnostics found material reality more pleasant, but still recognized the inviolable superiority of the soul and sought merger with the divine (Barnstone 1984: 368, 725–27; Ellwood 1983: 123). This trend culminated with theurgic Neoplatonism. Originally, the focus was on mediumistic trance and other orphic techniques. Later, in the fourth century theurgical Neoplatonism was influenced by the Chaldean/Egyptian approach of high magic and the summoning and control of godlings (Ellwood 1973: 52–54). The complilation of *Hermes Trismegistus*—a treatise on magic, astrology, and alchemy—made pagan gnosticism better known to Renaissance alchemists than Christian gnosticism.

At the same time, orthodox Christians and Greco-Romans of rationalist persuasion adhered to the idea of absolute truth, not dependent on personal revelation. In the Christian case, the authority of the church fathers was the source of this truth. For the pagan rationalists, philosophical mentors such as Aristotle and the deductions derived from material observation were the unchanging truth. Out of this school emerged Galen (A.D. 129–99), whose works became the standard for rationalist Hippocratic medicine (Coulter 1975: 217; Foster and Anderson 1978: 58). At the same time, the Neoplatonic Celsus (d. A.D. 185) denied the validity of the complex system of humors and perceived empiricism as the only logical approach in Roman medicine

(Coulter 1975: 241–57). In the third century, Celsus was followed by Sextus Empiricus, the last official Roman empirical physician. By the beginning of the fourth century, denying the authority of established truth was no longer fashionable or completely safe.

THE VEILED TRADITION

In A.D. 313, the Roman emperor Constantine decreed that Christianity, a particular orthodox brand, was the official religion of the empire. By the end of that century, heretics were endangered. The associated empirical medical tradition in Europe declined as a visible force. The focus shifted to Asia, and into the esoteric, sub-rosa, heretical traditions of Europe. The advantage of the decentralized social organization of the heretics permitted limited survival outside the visible institutions (Figure 4.4). The empirical tradition was to remain embedded in Christian and quasi-Christian mysticism until the thirteenth century.

In Asia, Chinese Buddhism experienced a golden age from the fourth through the ninth centuries. Pilgrimages to India from China reinforced pre-existing networks (Huard and Wong 1968: 84). Alchemical elixirs for longevity, if not immortality, passed from Taoism along the silk routes to Persia and Europe (Needham and Gwei-Djen 1969: 274). Once again, Persia became the center of European/Asian exchange. In A.D. 431, the Christian Nestorians were expelled from the formative Byzantine empire, bringing with them the flower of Greco-Roman medical texts, especially the rationalist works (Foster and Anderson 1978: 58; Filliozat 1964: 38). They missionized throughout Asia, and eventually the works they brought were translated into Arabic and Persian. The rise of Islam in the seventh century sent the Nestorians into obscurity, but the legacy of their naturalistic and rationalistic medicine was maintained in Moslem intellectual circles, in spite of occasional opposition from proponents of fundamentalist prophetic medicine (Bürgel 1976: 54–61). The explosion of Islam, however, did not halt the burgeoning silk trade from China to India, Persia, the Arabic world, and the Byzantine empire (Huard and Wong 1968: 31, 92).

From the seventh to the thirteenth centuries, the Islamic vector, even though internally diverse, like the Achaemenians and Hellenists before them, provided networks for exchange and revitalization across Asia. This eclectic reciprocity took place in an Asia increasingly dominated by Islam, during the seventh to eighth century. By the ninth cen-

FIGURE 4.4   A CHRONOLOGY OF THE EMPIRICAL MEDICAL TRADITION:
A.D. 301–1000, THE VEILED TRADITION

POLITICAL/ ECONOMIC HISTORY	PHILOSOPHICAL HISTORY	MEDICAL HISTORY
FOURTH CENTURY A.D.		
Europe: Christianity becomes official Roman religion A.D. 313		
China, India: A.D. 300–900 Golden Age of Chinese Buddhism, pilgrimages from China to India	China, Persia, Europe: fourth to sixth century Concepts of Im- mortality Elixers and alchemy diffuse from China by the silk routes to Europe	
FIFTH CENTURY A.D.		
	Europe, Persia: +431–850 Christian Nestorians expelled from Byzantine Empire, go to Persia, missionize in Asia, translate Greco- Roman medical works into Arabic	
SEVENTH CENTURY A.D.		
	Middle East: Islam is established	
China: Intensive trade relations with India, Persia, Arabic World, Byzantine Empire		
EIGHTH CENTURY A.D.		
Europe, Asia: Silk route to China flourishes; Islam expands		China, India, Middle East: Pulse diagnoses taught to India; Reciprocal exchange of materia medica

FIGURE 4.4 (*continued*)

POLITICAL/ ECONOMIC HISTORY	PHILOSOPHICAL HISTORY	MEDICAL HISTORY
NINTH CENTURY A.D.		
	Middle East: Moslem Sufi mysticism begins	Middle East, Persia: Translations are made of Greco-Roman medical texts; Rationalist physicians practice, Rhazes (860–932)
TENTH CENTURY A.D. India: Islam invades India A.D. 977–1200		

tury, Islam was revitalized by mystical Sufism and yet maintained rationalist Greco-Roman philosophy and medicine in Persia. Soon after, translations of Greek and Roman documents brought on a revival of Hippocratic doctrines (Foster and Anderson 1978: 58; Coulter 1975: 339). From the tenth to twelfth centuries, India was penetrated by Islam (Barraclough 1982: 40). Ayurvedic medicine faced a serious competitor in its sister tradition, now called Unani (Ionian or Greek) medicine. In the thirteenth century, Islamic geographers gave accounts of Chinese medicine that were to stimulate European interest centuries later (Needham 1970: 16).

The Crusades, from 1084–1204, devastated the remnants of the Byzantine Empire, but nonetheless reminded Europe of the rest of the Old World (see Figure 4.5). The crusading Palestinian Order of the Templars is virtually a mythological spring for European esoterica. Esoteric Freemasons of various kinds claim the Templars as their forefathers in a chain of secret knowledge flowing from the Holy Land (Addison 1978; see also Crow 1968: 170–71). This folk history is highly debatable but does demonstrate the repeated urge to create a traditional justification. It is common practice in esoteric circles to choose ones own ancestors. It also points out the value of the networks, however hostile, that were created in this era. By the fourth Crusade in the thirteenth

FIGURE 4.5 A CHRONOLOGY OF THE EMPIRICAL MEDICAL TRADITION:
A.D. 1001–1700, MYSTICAL REVIVALS

POLITICAL/ ECONOMIC HISTORY	PHILOSOPHICAL HISTORY	MEDICAL HISTORY
ELEVENTH CENTURY A.D.		
Europe, Middle East: Series of crusades invade Eastern Europe, Middle East through thirteenth century	Europe: The Free Spirit Movement begins	Persia: Avicenna (980–1036) writes *Canon of Medicine,* summing up known medical practices
TWELFTH CENTURY A.D.		
	Europe: twelfth and thirteenth century Gnostic Manichaean Albigensian revivals demonstrate Christian esoteric plurality, Spanish Moslems experience Sufi revival	Europe: Moorish and Judaic Spaniards pursue Galenic medicine, Avenzoar (1113–1162), Averroes (1126–1198), Moses ben Maimon (1135–1204)
THIRTEENTH CENTURY A.D.		
	Europe: Johannes Eckehart (1260–1329) (mystic) reintroduced Empiricist medicine; Mystical Judaic revival in Spain, Kabbalah tradition approaches, but does not espouse Neoplatonic divine mystical union	Middle East: Arabic geographers give accounts of Chinese medicine
SIXTEENTH CENTURY A.D.		
Europe: 1500–1900 European Expansion		Europe: Paracelsus (Philippus Aureolus) Theophrastus Bombast von Hohenheim (1493–1541) Mystic and catalyst for the Empirical paradigm, widely travelled

FIGURE 4.5 (continued)

POLITICAL/ ECONOMIC HISTORY	PHILOSOPHICAL HISTORY	MEDICAL HISTORY
SEVENTEENTH CENTURY A.D.		
	Europe: Rosicrucian Enlightenment (Protestant mysticism?); Georg Ernst Stahl (1660–1734) promotes the concept of vital essence	Europe: Dutch interest in Chinese medicine

century, trade advantages and political ties to the East were paramount concerns (Cohn 1970: 89).

Reciprocal exchange did ocur and influenced the course of religious, philosophical, and medical thought in Europe. Despite the clear institutional superiority of the Orthodox Roman Catholic Church, other religious practices, ecstatic and individualized, survived. The creation of Sufism in the ninth century is believed to be inspired by remnants of Christian heresy in the East. It, in turn, inspired the birth of the Free Spirit Movements in eleventh century Europe (Cohn 1970: 151–52). Christian Gnostic Manichaeans (a Christian/Zoroastrian/Buddhist synthesis), known as Albigensians, a strongly ascetic, dualistic group that denounced the impurity of matter, flourished briefly in twelfth and thirteenth century Europe (Prakash 1964: 248–49). The veiled tradition persisted.

The Free Spirit Movement, clearly an aspect of newly rediscovered Neoplatonism with a millenial vision, affected the Sufi resurgence in twelfth century Moorish Spain (Cohn 1970: 151–52). This in turn, probably influenced and was influenced by the thriving Kabbalistic tradition of Jewish mysticism. The Kabbalah took the concept of Neoplatonic merger with the divine, but stopped short, basking in, rather than joining, the divine light (Barnstone 1984: 142–43; Ellwood 1973: 55–56; Epstein 1978). Moorish Spain was the synthetic haven for rationalist as well as ecstatic concepts. Moorish and Jewish Spaniards revived rationalist medicine and reintroduced the works of Galen into European medical practice.

Empirical medicine again appeared as an open practice in thirteenth-century Europe through the efforts of Johannes Eckehart (1260–1329)—physician and mystic. He combined the two approaches to renovate empirical healing. Later, empiricism rose to new heights under the auspices of Phillipus Aureolus Theophrastus Bombast von Hohenheim (1493–1541), otherwise known as Paracelsus, (Coulter 1975: 339–483). He was a catalyst for the empirical tradition whose reach extended through time to such diverse thinkers as Carl Jung (Coulter 1975: 343), the Theosophist Blavatsky (Ellwood 1983: 121), and Randolph Stone of Polarity (1978: 19). Inspired by Neoplatonism, Paracelsus launched a one man attack on the rationalist schoolmen of the orthodox church, an act which led to his epithet, Prince of Charletans. He practiced his own heretical, millenarian brand of Christianity. Paracelsus was rumoured to belong to the Brethren of the Common Life, part of the Renaissance counterculture (Coulter 1975: 355). He castigated the authorities on medicine—Aristotle, Galen, and even Celsus, calling them "so many high asses" (Ellwood 1873: 59). Paracelsus doubted all authority (Ellwood 1973: 59) and naturally was despised by those authorities as a "bombastic" radical (Coulter 1975: 353–54).

He was thoroughly eclectic in his sources of medical knowledge, tapping the folk medicine of gypsies, miners, and "the wise" (Crow 1968: 208–9; Ellwood 1973: 59). He travelled widely and was reputed to have been captured by Tartars and entranced by their shamanistic practices. Paracelsus tested any remedy regardless of source. He refused to believe that practice followed vague theory and was staunchly empirical (Coulter 1975: 465). His eclectic experimentation led him to discover laudanum, perhaps to his detriment (Ellwood 1973: 59). He was an alchemist, and that meant his cosmological mechanisms were tied to esoteric Neoplatonism (Eliade 1976: 55). Paracelsus promoted the idea of "magnetism" as the mechanism by which the stars influence the microcosm, through the creative force that Paracelsus called imagination. Because the entire cosmos is interactive, separation of individual cause is impossible. Paracelsus promoted encyclopedic diagnostic techniques and sought the environmental factors that were critical to the empirical method.

Paracelsus advocated the idea of invoking bodily defense, an empirical concept fundamental to holistic health. He maintained that the physican may have limited knowledge of the cure, but the body will know how to heal itself if defended (Coulter 1975: 473). The idea of the body's innate intelligence as a living spirit seeking health can be seen in nearly all holistic health practices, especially chiropractic, homeopathy, and bodywork. It is conceptually akin to balancing ch'i and chakra energies.

Paracelsus lived in a rapidly expanding social environment. The Reformation had successfully challenged the established authority in church, science, and scholarship. European colonialism was beginning to stretch its political and economic tendrils into the Americas and Asia. By the seventeenth century, spurred by trade contacts, interest was renewed in imported medicine, and the Dutch began to publish accounts of Chinese medicine (Needham and Gwei-Djen 1980: 269). However, the Protestant Reformation may have removed some of the avenues for mystical expression that had been tolerated, barely, by Roman Catholicism. This is one explanation for the explosion of the seventeenth-century Rosicrucian Enlightenment (Crow 1978: 217). In 1614 the Order of the Rosy Cross, said to be founded by the magus Christian Rosenkreutz in the fourteenth century, advertised to bring new members into this secret society upon the receipt of treatises of mystical import. Many were sent, but the order remained silent. Impatient, some Englishmen founded their own society, later influencing Cambridge Neoplatonism and establishing an archetype for esoteric secret societies (Ellwood 1973: 60–62).

Empirical medicine remained alive, reanimated by the concept of *Anima sensitiva,* the vitalism of Georg Ernst Stahl (Coulter 1977: 60). Empirical medicine abandoned alchemy, the infant chemistry, initiated by Paracelsus and other empiricists, and concentrated primarily on elaborating the concept of vital essence (Coulter 1977: xv–xvi). The split between spiritual and materialist medicine grew sharper.

MASONS, MAGNETISM, SPIRITS AND SPAS

The Age of Reason, the eighteenth century, was also an age of mysticism in Europe and in the developing geographical center for metaphysics, America (see Figure 4.6). The German idealists, including Friedrich Hegel took the empirical concept of essence and expanded on it (Ellwood 1983: 122). Beginning in 1717 secret societies erupted, beginning in England. Isaac Newton was associated with the new Grand Lodge of England (Ellwood 1973: 62–64). The societies combined the archaic craft guild and the spirit of the Rosicrucian Enlightment, creating the sociological entity, the Freemasons (Ellwood 1983: 128). They ranged from mundane associations to hotbeds of esoterica. The Freemason phenomenon was associated with a mild anti-clerical deism, emphasizing moral deeds and echoing the idea of the distant diety of the Neoplatonists and Gnostics (Ahlstrom 1978: 13–18). The hallmark of the societies was their flair for ritual. Successful in England, Freemasonry was the darling of the new American elite. Whenever someone refers to the esoteric as un-American, I think of the Founding Fathers engaging in masonic Rosicrucian rites.

These organizations incorporated the bourgoisie and the elite and had political overtones. These "Illuminati," self ordained as enlightened beings, existed in Bavaria from 1776 to at least 1840. Adam Weishaupt and the Baron von Knigger modeled their masonic organization after the efficient Jesuits and infiltrated positions of power in Central Europe (Ellwood 1973: 64). They had radical antiroyalist sentiments, which may have contributed to the formative ideology of the French Revolution. Naturally, they were suppressed when their bias was discovered. They have been called pseudo-occult, "dreary materialists" by some (Crow 1968: 279). Their story does not stop in the past. Today the Illuminati are perceived as the masterminds for a continuing occult revolution by others, seriously and in jest (Wilson 1978; 1981). Their fundamental nature is always in doubt—neither clearly good nor evil. This aspect will be pursued again in chapter 5.

Concurrent with the Rosicrucian Enlightenment, the charismatic scientist Emanuel Svedberg, alias Swedenborg (1688–1772), influenced the shape of the estoeric in the eighteenth century. Swedenborg began to see visions consisting of trips through heaven and hell at the age of fifty-five. The philosophy he evolved was both Neoplatonic and based on personal revelation. He postulated the preexistence and postexistence of the soul and an invisible second coming, foreshadowing the intangible Aquarian dawn. He believed in the plurality of spheres and the continuation of God's consciousness with humanity's (Ellwood 1973: 65). Besides creating his own church of the New Jerusalem, he had profound influence in America.

American Spiritualism is a direct offspring, and transcendentalism

FIGURE 4.6   A CHRONOLOGY OF THE EMPIRICAL MEDICAL TRADITION:
A.D. 1700–1850, RATIONALIST PHYSICIANS,
SPIRITUALIST HEALERS

POLITICAL/ ECONOMIC HISTORY	PHILOSOPHICAL HISTORY	MEDICAL HISTORY
EIGHTEENTH CENTURY		
	Europe: German idealism, concern with essence; esoteric freemasonry born of guild and Rosicrucian Enlightenment; Bavarian Illuminati (1776–1840?) create republican political network; Anton Mesmer introduced animal magnetism; Emanuel Svedberg (Swedenborg 1688– 1772) creates mystical Christian Neoplato- nism, later develops into Spiritualism	Europe: Rise of state affiliated Rationalist medicine, church ties decline; the Age of Heroic Medicine-purging, bleeding, mercury elixirs in Rationalist medicine
	America: Freemasonry and Deism run rampant	

near kin, to Swedenborg's ideas. Spiritualism has been called the frontier application of Swedenborgianism (Ellwood 1973: 65). An American folk hero, Johnny Appleseed (John Chapman) was spreading Swedenborgian Spiritualism while wandering across America planting apple trees (Ellwood 1973: 65; 1979: 90). Meanwhile the Poughkeepsie Seer, Andrew Jackson Davis (1826–1910) launched American Spiritualism to new heights using the written word. Allan Kardec (Hyppolyte Leon Denizard Rivail [1801–1869]) promoted reincarnation, a minority posi-

FIGURE 4.6 *(continued)*

POLITICAL/ ECONOMIC HISTORY	PHILOSOPHICAL HISTORY	MEDICAL HISTORY
NINETEENTH CENTURY: 1800–1850		
Europe: Colonial expansion into India, Asia, Africa	Europe: Karl von Reichenbach (1788–1869) creates concept of the Odic force, the vital essence	Europe: Samuel Hahnemann (1755–1843) creates homeopathy, combining medicine and Neoplatonism
America: Political and geographic expansion	America: New England Transcendentalism (1830s); Phineas Quimby (1802–1866), founds New Thought; Andrew Jackson Davis, the Poughkeepsie Seer (1826–1910), promotes American Spiritualism as does John Chapman (Johnny Appleseed 1774–1845).	America: Constantine Hering promotes homeopathy in 1835; Samuel Thomson (1755–1843) creates an herbal healing movement; Wooster Beach (1794–1859) creates the Eclectic school synthesizing homeopathy and Thomsonian herbalism; Sylvester Graham (1794–1851) creates health food movement; American Medical Association is founded in response to Empiricists

tion in nineteenth-century American Spiritualism (Ellwood 1973: 73–74). Although this movement supposedly peaked in 1850 and passed into obscurity, holistic health seekers still "visualize" spirit guides and wander through different planes of reality in a self-hypnotic state of "altered consciousness." The terminology differs, but the legacy is clearly Spiritualist.

Spiritualism was not Swedenborg's only American endowment. The naturalistic New England transcendentalists, Thoreau and Whitman, owed much to both Swedenborg and the rediscovery of the East (Albanese 1977; Koster 1975: 5–6; Ellwood 1983: 127). The transcendentalists influenced such diverse movements as New Thought, Theosophy (Ellwood 1979: 84), and the Dharma Bums (American Buddhists of the late 1950s). American transcendentalism and German idealism combined to produce New Thought (Ellwood 1983: 122). Born with the catalyst Phineas Quimby (1802–1866), New Thought held that mind is "fundamental and causative" (Ellwood 1973: 79). New Thought produced Unity, Religious Science, and the Church of Divine Science, among a host of smaller organizations. New Thought reified nineteenth-century American optimism. In its purest form, this optimism rejoiced that anything was possible with the help of the "Universal Mind" (Koster 1975: 85–87). The healing and conversion of a young invalid, Mary Baker Eddy, by Quimby, led to another interpretation of New Thought (Freedland 1972: 65) and the birth of Christian Science in 1866. Eddy maintained that it was misleading to ask the Mind for aid, when actually the grace was already there and illness was only an illusion (Freedland 1972: 65). Christian Science epitomized the direction empirical healing was taking in the eighteenth and nineteenth centuries (Ahlstrom 1978: 17). A clear division developed between self-responsibility/ spirituality and orthodox medicine.

Rationalist medicine developed new features. Medicine had been tightly associated with the church. During the eighteenth century French orthodox medicine began to disassociate from the church and align itself with the increasingly powerful state. Radical new ideas, such as conceptually treating disease as an entity, rather than treating a "diseased person" came into being (Treacher and Wright 1982: 3–4; Foucault 1973: 14, 118–19). Even the teaching methods changed. Instead of the traditional combination of theoretical learning and apprenticeship, medical arts were taught at a clinical school (Foucault 1973). Along with this standardized training came a new thrust toward professionalism. Orthodox medicine was structurally transformed.

From 1780 to 1850, orthodox medicine suffered through the Age of Heroic Medicine. This "heroism" referred to the measures practiced to stamp out disease. Violent purging, the use of calomel—mercurous oxide—and bleeding made heroes of the survivors (Coulter 1973: 5; Duffy 1979; Kaufman 1971: 1–4). The inappropriate extention of useful remedies to other ailments and the excessive use of major therapies had "the appearance of institutionalized folly" (Thomas 1981).

Empirical medicine was a direct response to this situation. The works of F. Anton Mesmer (1734–1815) (Ellwood 1983: 122), and later Karl von Reichenbach (1788–1869) provided a backdrop for the idea of healing through animal magnetism and the odic force (named after Odin, the Norse god [Crow 1968: 299]). If vital forces could be invoked to defend the body, lethal doses of mercury would not be necessary. Samuel Hahnemann (1755–1843) developed homeopathy in the belief that "the native army could defeat the enemy with the help of auxilliary troops" (Kaufman 1971: 25–26). Homeopathy used minute doses of substances that produced symptoms similar to the ailment. The remedies were "potentiated" so that the spiritual essence of the remedy could work on the spiritual body. Belief in the doctrine of correspondences—the link between the microcosm and the macrocosm—was essential to this practice. Swedenborgianism and transcendentalism made plural spiritual planes more comprehensible to common folk (Kaufman 1971: 25–26). In addition, Hahnemann's empiricism and careful record of his experiments were superior to most efforts among his materialist contemporaries.

Homeopathy made its way to America in the 1830s, promoted by Constantine Hering (Duffy 1979: 114; Kaufman 1971: 28). Although Hering developed a homeopathic home remedy kit, it remained a professional healing technique (Numbers 1977: 59). Homeopathic doctors were still necessary for diagnosis and proper prescription. This distinguished homeopathy from other empirical healing practices that developed in the nineteenth century. Samuel Thomson (1755–1843), learned in grassroots herbalism, advocated self care and scorned professional interference (Numbers 1977: 55). However, his herbal lore was soon taken up by students who made it more systematic and professional (Duffy 1979: 112). Sylvester Graham (1794–1851) of cracker fame, prescribed the use of whole grain foods, fresh air, and exercise as superior healing techniques (Duffy 1979: 119–21). In the vein of empirical professionals, Wooster Beach (1794–1859) joined herbalism, naturalism, and homeopathy together and created "Eclecticism," a foreshadowing of naturopathy (Duffy 1979: 114).

The end of the Age of Heroic medicine and the beginning of rationalist professionalism came in 1850. In 1847, orthodox medicine responded to the professional erosion brought on by empirical medicine and formed the American Medical Association. Although many of the A.M.A. physicians were sympathetic to the aims and beliefs of the empiricists, they realized the empiricists were a threat to professional survival. Excluding empiricals from positions of governmental importance, hospital work, and professional organizations, the A.M.A. became the wedge that formally split empirical and rationalist medicine in the nineteenth century (Duffy 1979: 117–19).

Natural and spiritual medicine were not easily dismissed (see Figure 4.7). Travelling practitioners with a wide range of expertise and charisma amused and educated American citizens in the second half of the nineteenth century (Freedland 1972: 62). Each town, including Paraiso, had its lyceum, a lecture hall where homeopaths and speakers, such as Paraiso's "Queen of Magnetism," an electropath and spiritualist medium, lectured and gathered clients (Baur 1959: 89). By the 1880s, naturalist health spas and resorts had become the fashionable response to chronic illness. "Watering places" in Europe formed havens of empirical healing. Southern California began to be known as the ideal environment for taking the airs, drinking the waters, and consuming healthy fresh fruits and vegetables. Four areas emerged as centers of natural cure, including Paraiso (Baur 1959). In 1873, Charles Nordhoff, booster extraordinary, wrote *California for Travelers and Settlers,* serialized in *Harper's Magazine,* praising Paraiso as the world's ideal health resort (Hill 1930; Tompkins 1975: 55–56). The editor of the local paper launched an advertising campaign for all of southern California, but specifically exalting Paraiso (Baur 1959: 66). Up to a hundred health seekers would invade Paraiso, with each new steamboat (Baur 1959: 67; Hill 1930). Many were prominent bourgeois Easterners and Europeans, which contributed to the image of Paraiso as a more refined and cultured place than neighboring resorts. It became known as the haven of the "wealthy and unhealthy" (Baur 1959: 69). One enthusiastic citizen wrote,

> Fair Paraiso, to thee
> Is given a sacred ministry.
> To thee the sick and suffering
> Their hopes and fears and sorrows bring.
> Would those sad hearts so sorely tried,
> Might see their longing satisfied!
> (Baur 1959: 18–19, originally written 1878)

Enticing these ailing emigrants, one Paraiseño physician claimed that the "oleaginous fumes" that occasionally loomed over the area

FIGURE 4.7   A CHRONOLOGY OF THE EMPIRICAL MEDICAL TRADITION:
1851–1900, SPAS AND SPIRITS

POLITICAL/ ECONOMIC HISTORY	PHILOSOPHICAL HISTORY	MEDICAL HISTORY
NINETEENTH CENTURY: 1851–1900		
Europe: Colonial expansion intensifies in India, Asia, and Africa	Europe: Order of the Golden Dawn established on Rosicrucian lines, includes MacGregor Mathers (brother-in-law of Henri Bergson), Aleister Crowley	Europe: Spas become fashionable health centers
America: America adopts a policy of manifest destiny after the civil war, immigration of diverse elements continues	America: California attracts utopian colonists, Spiritualist community established near Paraiso 1883; Mary Baker Eddy founds Christian Science 1866 out of New Thought doctrines; Helena Petrovna Blavatsky (1831–1891) founds Theosophy circa 1888 with Colonel Henry Olcott; World Parliament of Religions held in Chicago 1893 and Vedanta Societies of philosophical Hinduism are founded	America: Osteopathy is created in the 1870s; Palmer creates chiropractic 1895; Southern California becomes major center for health resorts; Paraiso is one of four prime areas, booms from 1870– 1900

were actually curative (Baur 1959: 9; Tompkins 1975: 56). Hot springs were discovered from the 1850s to the 1870s. Near Paraiso, several companies bottled the water and sold it throughout Southern California. Paraiseño's mineral water was considered the best in the United States and comparable to European waters (Baur 1959: 102). Coupled with the Mediterranean climate, Paraiso rapidly became an international watering place.

Paraiso's reputation as a gigantic spa was supplanted by tourism by the twentieth century, but the health resort image remains imbedded in Paraiseño ethos. Other historical factors contributed to Paraiso's attraction to empirical medicine. Nineteenth- and early twentieth-century California was attractive to those pursuing the esoteric as well as to the seekers of well-being and longevity.

COLONIALISM'S
UNACKNOWLEDGED LEGACY

In the late nineteenth and early twentieth century, California attracted utopian settlers and colonists (Hine 1983). Some sought communities in which they could pursue inner knowledge, unhindered by outside interference. A neighboring village of Paraiso became a flourishing home for Spiritualists in the 1880s and 1890s (Lathim and Lathim 1975: 10–49). By the 1920s health spas in Camino Robles existed side by side with centers for the advancement of revealed mystical knowledge. The Theosophical center, Krotona, named after. the ancient Pythagorean school, synthesized concepts from Tibet, China, India, Egypt, and Hellenistic Europe.

This eclecticism would not have been possible without the European colonial expansion into Africa, India, and Asia (see Figures 4.7 and 4.8). Europeans and Americans could see for themselves the wonders of the Orient, hear about them through travelling lecturers and tourists, and read about them. The esoteric is a literary phenomenon. If mentors were not available in person, their words were accessible through the printed page. Publications of primary sources were available, such as the gnostic text *Pistis Sophia,* translated in 1851. Others excavated in Egypt were printed in 1884. In 1909, Manichaean texts were found in Turkestan. The Essene Dead Sea scrolls from Qumran and the Nag Hammadi gnostic texts added to the fervor in the twentieth century (Walker 1983; 26–27). The meeting of the World Parliament of Religions in Chicago in 1893, led to the creation of the Vedanta societies, which spread philosophical Hinduism (Ellwood 1973: 81).

Eclectic syntheses, such as Theosophy (see Ellwood 1983) and the Order of the Golden Dawn, were the primary vehicles for the dissemination of imported ideas. Theosophy, divine wisdom, was founded

FIGURE 4.8   A CHRONOLOGY OF THE EMPIRICAL MEDICAL TRADITION:
1901–1960, THE STAGE IS SET

POLITICAL/ ECONOMIC HISTORY	PHILOSOPHICAL HISTORY	MEDICAL HISTORY
1901–1960		
The World: First and Second World Wars and the breakdown of political colonialism	Europe: Anthroposophy founded by Rudolf Steiner (1861–1925) from Neoplatonism and Theosophy, oriented toward healing; Carl Gustav Jung (1875–1961) develops a school of psychology in the 1920–1930s that draws on the work of Paracelsus and Chinese mysticism	
	America: Edgar Cayce (1847–1945), practices psychic healing and develops doctrine of Christian reincarnation and karma; Theosophy spawns a series of new groups—the Rosicrucian Fellowship (1907), a healing order; Katherine Tingley's Universal Brotherhood of Theosophy at Pt. Loma (until 1942); Annie Besant's Esoteric Theosophical and Krotona Institutes at Camino Robles, as well as Alice Bailey's Esoteric Studies Publicity Center	India, China: Reactionary governments discourage traditional medicine; this process is reversed after colonial independence and traditional Indian, and especially Chinese medicine are revitalized

by the charismatic Madame Helena Petrovna Blavatsky (1831–1891) and her collegue, Colonel Henry Olcott. The eccentric Blavatsky travelled for many years seeking secret knowledge and incorporating her understanding of Oriental mysteries and personal revelations. Olcott and Blavatsky started their work in Spiritualist circles and later travelled to India in the 1880s. Her book *The Secret Doctrine* began a literary movement augmented by her charismatic personality (Ellwood 1973: 93). Her delight in things Oriental and her use of revealed knowledge, spoken through trances, created allies, opponents, and mimics. Her one-time follower, Rudolf Steiner (1861–1925), disagreed that India and Tibet were the sources of special knowledge and fostered the return to Christian gnostic and Neoplatonic sources (Steiner 1973: 47; Ellwood 1973: 100–108). Steiner also maintained that trance-revealed information should be accessible to the public and that the process should be studied openly and with minimal mystery (Ellwood 1973: 28). With these ideas he founded Anthroposophy in Europe, a school with healing applications. After Blavatsky's death in 1891, Theosophy split into rival schools. One, centered on William Judge and Katherine Tingley, ultimately led to a utopian community called Point Loma. The other, continued by Olcott and then by C. W. Leadbeater and Annie Besant, led to the 1924 opening of Krotona in Camino Robles, the esoteric heart of Theosophy (Freedland 1972: 71; Ellwood 1973: 100).

Theosophy, like second-century gnosticism, revolved around revealed truth. Truth was gained through personal insight, experience, and communication with the spirit planes and the unconscious. Particularly after Freud and Jung legitimized the idea that the unconscious could convey coherent meaning, dreams and trances could be seen as more than mere chaos (Eliade 1976: 53). The implication, as the early Christians had learned to their distress, is that anyone could be the recipient of revealed knowledge. The early twentieth century rang with new revelations of cosmological and religious truths. Among the most important for healing were Edgar Cayce (Freedland 1972: 198–201; McGarey 1978: 199) and Alice Bailey (1980; Ellwood 1973: 103). Cayce had been influenced by Theosophy (Ellwood 1978: 269) and Bailey had been an active member until her own visions became too prominent. Both practiced and taught psychic healing and emphasized the importance of reincarnation and the spiritual second coming of Christ. The Rosicrucian Fellowship, a Theosophical spinoff founded by Max

Heindel (Carl Louis van Grasshoff) in 1907, also focuses on healing and astrology (Ellwood 1973: 111). Cayce, Bailey, and the Rosicrucian Fellowship have all played a part in the conceptions of holistic health practitioners in Paraiso, along with the metaphysicists of the Order of the Golden Dawn.

The Order of the Golden Dawn was part of the English Freemason tradition. Especially inspired by Egyptian archaeology, the members dabbled in trance, tarot, and theurgy. One leader, MacGregor Mathers was the brother-in-law of the French philosopher Henri Bergson (Crow 1968: 285), who elaborated on elan vital, the vital force (Bergson 1913: 42). One of their stars, later to form his own order, was a magus of dubious moral fiber, Aleister Crowley. The ambiguity and mystery of his character added to his charisma. Like the Illuminati (with their questionable morality), he is the source of myth and color in the Aquarian movement. He is the trickster, the Aquarian counterpoint to the Afro-American Anansi and Native American coyote who cannot be trusted, but may reveal truth and give help (Crow 1968: 287–290; Wilson 1978; 1981).

As some Europeans and Americans were seeking the knowledge of the Orient, others were doing their best to educate the East into the ways of "Western Civilization." The postdynastic Chinese government (Wang 1979: 301) and the British (Montgomery 1976: 276; Sanyal 1964: 11) discouraged the practice of traditional Chinese and Ayurdevic medicine. The nationalism of Gandhi's independence movement and especially the Maoist revolution in China accented this issue and made it legitimate to practice naturalistic medicine again. New books were published. Texts that had been lost were regained in China and new editions were printed of classic works (Porkert 1976: 76). A concerted effort was made in China to systematize the diverse family traditions and create a new profession, competitive and cooperative with orthodox medicine. Ayurvedic medicine, although less successful than the Chinese in this regard, also formed colleges and institutions to aid professionalization. Homeopathy, introduced into India in 1839 (Sanyal 1964: 181), was philosophically compatable with the Ayurveda (see Leslie 1976: 359). Scorned by orthodox medicine, homeopaths were not hampered by the stigma of imperialism. Syntheses produced between the Ayurveda and homeopathy show up on the streets of Paraiso. The nationalism fomented by the end of political colonialism in China and

India, fostered a new period of eclecticism and exchange within the naturalistic, empirical medical systems.

THE PROTEAN PRACTITIONER

Trading linkages, conquests, and missionary efforts—by Buddhists, Christians, Moslems, and Manichaeans—created networks of exchange. In our era, society has seen Gandhi's nonviolent resistance on the streets of Tennessee and aspirin in the heart of Surinam's tropical forest. Historically, this exchange of concepts and materia medica periodically waxed and waned. The key to the empirical tradition has been a legacy of revealed and changing truths, characterized by the superiority of the spirit and an impatience with orthodox authority. The colonial expansion of Rome, Islam, and modern Europe created the opportunity for the exchanges of information between empirical traditions. Cultural contact created an ambiguity that promoted the desire for orthodox authority on one hand and created a niche for changing truth on the other. Contact and change gave birth to both the gnostic and authoritarian strategies.

Robert Ellwood, social historian of the new religions, refers to the formation of "Protean Man," whose spiritual life is not tied to a monolithic cultural identity but is changing and based on individual experience (1973: 299; 1983a: 121). This adaptability, he suggests, produced the Protean person. He ties this to a continuous tradition of alternative altars in Europe from the time of Pythagoras (Ellwood 1973: 42–84). This plasticity, the ability to mold to altering conditions, has been seen periodically throughout recorded history, relying on decentralized networks, bound by changing ideas and individual charisma. Ellwood traces the tradition of the mage to the concept of "shaman-in-civilization." What must not be overlooked is that in addition to being a religious leader, the shaman is a healer. The empirical medical tradition in healing is an another aspect of the shaman-in-civilization. An anthropologist must ask how groups without centralization maintain a cultural tradition during the reign of orthodoxy. In chapter 5, I explore the social movement as the medium of its survival.

THE GOALS OF HOLISTIC HEALTH

You know, we had gone to the hospital to see my mother, and I'd been in to see her, and I saw this woman that looked as bad as any survivor of Auschwitz or Dachau, and I was out in the hall sort of comforting my father, and this doctor who was a specialist in a problem that she had with her arm went into her room and came out just beaming and said to us, "Boy don't we have a lot of reason to feel great? Isn't that wonderful *how she's coming along?" Well, all he saw was her arm. That's all he saw . . . the moment before, we saw somebody who looked already dead, and now here comes the specialist who tells us that everything is great . . . uh, you know, you can go crazy.* (My Dinner with Andre, Shawn and Gregory 1981: 61–62)

Where is the holistic health movement going? People are not coming all the way from New Jersey or Seattle to Paraiso just to amuse themselves with a novel sense of communitas. Novices sitting day after day in a stuffy holistic academy, those living in Polarity Fellowships, or attending Esalen style workshops are there for a reason. If the social movement is goal-directed, purposeful behavior, what is the aim?

Proceeding from the general to the specific, I begin the exploration of this question with the process of social movements. Although any social movement consist of individuals, how do they act as systems? If a social movement is a subsystem of the larger cultural collectivity, then change must follow patterns common to all complex systems. Catastrophe theory and hierarchical restructuring provide analogies that help to reveal such patterns and can be used to illuminate the process of sudden changes within complex systems.

Success or failure is the critical issue in any adaptive scenario. Observers must accurately determine the hierarchy of goals in a social movement. Primary goals are ideological, binding the people to a common purpose. Implementing the goals, however, produces a secondary set of institutional goals. It is possible that the secondary goals may usurp the primary ones. In the traditional Weberian model of institutionalization, the shift to the mainstream of society is the climax. Does this mean that the secondary survival goals have transcended the original ones? If so, how is success determined?

This abstract exploration is a prelude to a concrete review of the cycle of a social movement, the skeleton framework of this entire ethnography. Where does the holistic health movement fit into this framework as a social phenomenon? As a vehicle of change, movements have a dynamic relationship with the culture. What aspect of the culture gives the social movement its power to transform? Ideology is the key. I am not implying the existence of only one ideology or one supportive organization. The diversity of beliefs and corresponding social structures are hallmarks of social movements, especially in the early stages. A summary of the various "catalytic analyses" in holistic health quickly illustrates the connections and segmentations within the field (see Figures 5.1, 5.2). These segmentations are bound together by similar visions of a transformative future.

The direction of the future is the prominent feature of the diverse teachings of leading figures in holistic health. The most fascinating aspect to emerge is the apparent underlying theme of global transformation, linking the specific movement of holistic health to the broader

FIGURE 5.1   A SAMPLE OF MAJOR CATALYTIC ANALYSES SINCE 1830

Primary Analysts (created major schools of thought
or spread fundamental ideas)

ANALYST	FIELD	COMMENTS
1830–1860		
Samuel Hahnemann	Homeopathy	Influenced Vithoulkas
Samuel Thomson	Herbalism	Influenced Jensen and Christopher
Phineas Quimby	Faith Healing	Taught Mary Baker Eddy, Evans
1861–1880		
Mary Baker Eddy	Christian Science	Healed by Quimby
Warren Evans	New Thought Churches	Student of Quimby
Madam Blavatsky/ H. Olcott	Theosophical movement	Influenced Bailey and Cayce
Matthias Alexander	Movement therapy	Resonates with Feldenkreis
N. Liljequist	Iridology	Influenced Jensen
Andrew Still	Osteopathy	Influenced Palmer
1881–1900		
Ignatz von Peczely	Iridology	Influenced Jensen
Daniel Palmer	Chiropractic	Student of Still
Nicola Tesla	Electro-magnetism	Influenced Kirlians
1901–1920		
William Fitzgerald	Zone Therapy-reflexology	Influenced Stone
Rudolph Steiner	Anthroposophical Medicine	Influenced Moss
1921–1940		
Randolph Stone	Polarity	Taught Pannetier and Campbell
Carl Jung	East/West Philosophical Syntheses	Influenced innovative psychologists, used Paracelsus and Asian Medicine

FIGURE 5.1 (*continued*)

ANALYST	FIELD	COMMENTS
1941–1960		
Wilhelm Reich	Orgone (vital force) therapy	"Father of holistic health," taught Rolf, Lowen, Kelly
Moshe Feldenkreis	Movement therapy	Influenced Aston Patterning
Tokujiro Namikoshi	Shiatsu	Influenced bodyworkers
Jiro Murai	Jin Shin Jitsu	Taught Teeguardens
1961–1980		
George Ohsawa	Macrobiotics	
Fernand Lamaze	Natural Childbirth (1950's)	

vision of the new age, Aquarian goals. A section of this chapter will elaborate on that topic.

Finally, a comparative perspective is fundamental in cultural anthropology. To this end, I employ an analysis of the early phases of another social movement, Christianity. Its duration, initial diversity, and detail of documentation make it an appropriate analogue. In addition, as chapter 4 illustrated, the history of mystical Christianity is intimately linked with the antecedents of Aquarian ideology.

THE CYBERNETIC SOCIAL MOVEMENT

Culture is a highly complex phenomenon. Analytically, everything is linked to all other components. This is what is meant by the classic phrase from introductory cultural anthropology that "Culture is integrated." The best analogy I know for this is a Rubik's cube, the toy that consists of a cube with nine squares on each of the six sides. Each square is one of six colors. The object is to have only one color for all nine cells on each side. This simple goal is exceedingly difficult to achieve. One reason for this complexity is that no single colored cell can be isolated. Each time the cube is manipulated to move one cell to its appropriate position, other squares are changed. To solve the puzzle,

FIGURE 5.2   A SAMPLE OF MAJOR CONSTRUCTIVE ANALYSES

Constructive Analysts—Implemented Primary Analyses
and created New Schools

ANALYST	FIELD	COMMENTS
1920–1940		
Edward Bach	Bach Flower Remedies	Applies homeopathic principles to flowers and emotions
Edgar Cayce	Psychic Healing	
Semyon and Valentina Kirlian	Electro-magnetism	Influenced by Tesla
Jethro Kloss	Herbalism	Author of *Back to Eden*
1941–1960		
Bernard Jensen	Iridology	
Alice Bailey	Psychic Healing	Author of "Esoteric" Healing
Marian Chace	Dance Therapy	
1961–1980		
George Vithoulkas	Homeopathy	
Charles Kelley	Radix (Neo-Reichian)	Student of Reich
Alexander Lowen	Bioenergetics (Neo-Reichian)	Student of Reich
Arthur Pauls	Orthobionomy	
Robert Whiteside	Personology (Physiognomy)	
John Christopher	Herbology	
Adele Davis, Nathan Pritikin*	Nutritional therapy	
Linus Pauling*	Orthomolecular Medicine	
Fritz Perls, Aldous Huxley, A. Maslow, Alan Watts, Carl Rogers, Rollo May	Created Esalen (1960s) and Humanistic Psychology	Influenced by Reich and Jung
Ida Rolf	Structural Integration	Student of Reich, Feldenkreis

FIGURE 5.2   (*continued*)

ANALYST	FIELD	COMMENTS
Mary Whitehouse*	Dance Therapy	
Judith Aston*	Aston Patterning, Movement Therapy	Student of Rolf
Jefferson Campbell*	Polarity	Student of Stone
Pierre Pannetier	Polarity	Student of Stone
John Christopher	Herbology and Cleansing	
Fritjof Capra*	New Age Physics	
Jane Roberts	Psychic Phenomena	Author of "Seth" books
Rosalyn Bruyere	Psychic Healing	
Thelma Moss	Psychic Phenomena	
Richard Bach	New Age Consciousness	Author of New Age Fiction
Thea Alexander	New Age Consciousness	Author of New Age Fiction
Joan Halifax*	Shamanistic Consciousness	Anthropological synthesist
Jean Houston	Innovative Psychology	
Norman Cousins*	Laughter Therapy, Behavioral Medicine	
Dolores Krieger	Therapeutic Touch	Applies energetic healing to Nursing
Kenneth Pelletier*	Holistic Medicine	
Ron and Iona Teeguarden*	Jin Shin Do	Students of Jiro Murai
Wataru Ohashi*	Zen Shiatsu	
George Goodheart, Paul Thie	Touch for Health	Synthesized chiropractic, acupressure

Visited Paraiso during the study period

seemingly irrelevant steps must be taken long before the actual fruition. Tracing the puzzle of causation is mind boggling.

Tracking the initial causational twists of a social movement involves playing with a vast conceptual Rubik's cube. Decisions made in the second century are relevant to the choices made by the local psychic healer in Paraiso, one cell in the holistic health movement. A cold that will not go away, a motorcycle accident, or a rude doctor at a father's death bed may change the course of an individual life and the movement at large. There is a map, however, for conceptualizing this process. It is catastrophe theory.

Catastrophe theory models the sudden jump of a system following a set of gradually changing circumstances (Zeeman 1982: 316–17). It is no wonder that the histories of holistic health start in 1960, as if the movement "appeared from nowhere." The long history of individual critical decisions were virtually invisible to the casual observer. Only the change, the hierarchical restructuring, was noticable. Shifting the time scale to a larger frame of reference, the chain of developments appears as a continuous tradition (Platt 1970: 53). The stream of events described in chapter 4 resembles a continuous change. Changing the perspective to a smaller time frame, sudden shifts become visible (Platt 1970: 53). Each historical jump—the concept of a separate soul, the idea of vital essence, the development of elemental and energetic naturalistic medical theories—is a sudden shift when viewed separately.

In the catastrophe model, the initial state of the system is in flux, not static. Over time, the change was preceeded by others, and will be followed by yet more. The overall appearance is that of a continuous stream of events. The shift comes at a critical point of divergence. Events can go in at least two directions. Each direction limits the process to a specific pattern. The sudden shift of that pattern is the "catastrophe." After the catastrophe, the pattern restructures itself and becomes a new form (see Platt 1970 for an explanation of hierarchical restructuring). This process is illustrated in Figure 5.3. In the illustration, the medical tradition of the nineteenth century is used as an example. The medical system of that century was in flux. Both empirical and rationalist medical systems were functional. How did they diverge? "Naturalism"—the promotion of noninvasive, natural remedies—was one of the many issues separating the two approaches. It was a point at which the empirical physicians supporting naturalism rapidly diverged from their rationalist colleagues. The sudden jump, the "catastrophe," reformed the beliefs and practices of nineteenth-century empirical medicine. The tradition continued to be shaped by other issues—spiritualism, vital force, resurgence of manipulative arts (chiropractic, osteopathy), and the concepts of homeopathy.

The process of continuity, jump, and reformation has interesting implications for the study of social movements. In this model, the past

FIGURE 5.3   A MODEL OF CATASTROPHE AND HEIRARCHICAL RESTRUCTURING
                 EXAMPLE: DIVERGENCE IN THE NINETEENTH CENTURY MEDICAL
                 TRADITION

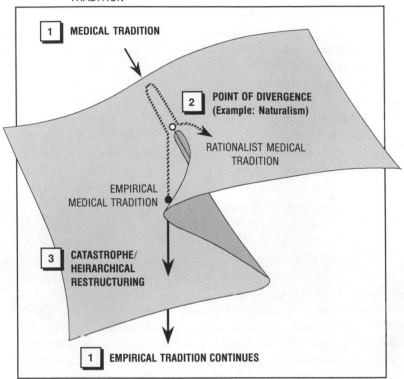

and the future of the movement are dynamic, not fixed (Zeeman 1977: 41, 344, 347). This understanding parallels the axiom in systems theory that complex systems are usually failing (Gall 1975: 61), never achieving balance and goal. Contrast this approach with a starting point of homeostasis. Change is more like reality. Each system has factors that limit the path of choice to several defined directions prior to the shift. In other words, once the point of schism is reached, the system may go two ways. Each way has its own set of reinforcements that push the system one way or another. This model can be used to organize thoughts about fission at a societal scale, for example, between orthodox and alternative medical systems. It can also be used within a social movement as a metaphor for the shift to empirical professional, underground healer, and for future syntheses in holistic health. The catastrophe model also makes a distinction between events influenced by immediate local conditions and those shaped by long term global conditions (Zeeman 1977: 308; 1982: 321–23). This discussion sets the stage for the examination of social traps—a situation in which short term advantages lead to long term disadvantages. What decisions—made on the basis of local information—ultimately inhibit adaptation to global conditions? The decision to react to local institutions may sap the movement of its original enthusiasm. What, then, determines the success or failure of a movement?

A Spencerian legacy has impeded the understanding of social movements in cultural evolution. A "survival of the fittest" mentality pervades the sociological and anthropological literature on social movements. Because of it, social scientists have difficulty in evaluating the real impact of social movements on the culture. Social scientists have not only been asking the wrong question of social movements, we also lack the tools to evaluate success and failure. Without this baseline, we cannot transcend the notion that social movements are merely interesting phenomena of deviance. Are these the only alternatives?

My tirade has two points. First, in a mature ecosystem, adaptation requires stability and diversity, not merely productivity (Odum 1966: 88). In the social sciences, however, a "majority rule" concept seems to dictate the definition of success or failure in a social movement. The "goal" of adaptation, by their definition, is ecological climax, the creation of the maximally stable system. Climax ecosystems are not simple, but are composed of diverse species and a wealth of niches (Odum 1966: 85). Human ecosystems are also diverse. This diversity is no more abnormal than it is abnormal to have manzanita in a Yellow Pine forest. Every plant in the forest does not have to be a pine to achieve adaptive success for pines. The fact that something else exists besides manzanita, does not make the shrub a "failure." Come the next forest fire, it will be valuable in the habitat.

Pushing the analogy to its limits, human diversity provides potential for the society. Majority rule is not the only criterion for success. If every social movement does not become the Roman Catholic Church, does that imply failure? Church and movement do not occupy the same niche. The underground religious movement may not even be competing with the Catholic Church. The two may coexist. A contrary position has crept into social scientific thinking. The assumption has been that if the social movement has not quickly institutionalized, then it was just a deviant flash in the pan. Institutionalization—the Weberian routinization of individual charisma—has been the traditional baseline for "success" (Ash and Zald 1969: 472).

Second, social movements do not spring from a "steady state." No culture is ever "finished and homeostatic." The conceptual model of homeostasis parallels ecological climax, but it is subtly different. In zealous moments, social scientists (including me, at times) seem to think this process ends. No biologist worth his paycheck would assume the climax of an ecological succession was the final state of the system. However, even the most elegant models of social movements may begin and end with the words "steady state" (Wallace 1956: 268), implying maximum institutionalization. This kind of premise changes the way in which dissonance is perceived. If there is a final adaptation, then dissonance is an unusual condition. If there is no real final solution, then perhaps dissonance is a phenomenon of living systems, not a prime mover.

I am not abusing an ethnographic dead horse. I am frequently asked by colleagues and students, "Why study these wierdos who are not satisfied with the best medical system in the world but are only adopting faddish foreign ways?" Somehow, studying American culture brings out hidden ethnocentrism. The implication is that the perceptions of the holistic health participants are unjustified; they do not represent the majority opinion and therefore lie outside the American experience. American culture, like any system, is always in flux. The diversity that gave birth to holistic health existed long before the movement was given its name. That diversity is the key to the role a social movement plays in cultural adaptation.

My critical task was to identify the nature of this diversity. The practitioners of holistic health are not ethnically, linguistically, or phenotypically distinct. They have mothers and cats, pay bills, watch movies, and live quite like other Americans. What makes them discrete? Their beliefs, practices, and frequently decentralized organizations give them their unique niche.

Ideology supports the adaptive mechanisms of technology, economics, and social organization by providing values that justify the existence of institutions and create a blueprint for future behavior. Ideology serves to filter out the perceptions of alternatives and justifies the behavior based on these perceptions. It provides the cognitive environment in which humans must function. This understanding of ideology is similar to the concepts of the social and physical environments, the cultural manifestations of social organization and economy. Ideology is a learned behavior complex, analogous to instinct in animals except that it interacts with culture rather than genetic programming, and is probabilistic, not deterministic. Ideology is the culturewide and culture specific codification of behavioral guides. Much as natural selection acts on the codification of genetically based behavior, social reinforcement acts on cultural behavior. If a behavior works, or does not, the ideology that generated it is reinforced, positively or negatively. The trick is to know what is working, and what only appears to be working in the short term. This is difficult to observe in a complex system, where any failure may be hidden from view (Gall 1975: 54).

I propose that adaptive success should be defined more widely than mere Weberian institutionalization. Social movements can, indeed, be viewed in a different light. Not all stable social movements look like the Catholic Church. After all, the Christian esoteric tradition has coherently existed for an equally long period of time, without necessarily adopting a cohesive institutional framework. This perspective minimizes the red herring effect of deviance and majority adaptation as definitions of failure and success. Perhaps minority ideas are a "real" part of the complexity of culture, just as manzanita and malodorous mountain misery are a critical part of Yellow Pine forest ecology.

Having tilted at the windmill, I must still provide some redefinition of success. For evaluation alone, I suggest that any system that can reproduce its own primary goals, the ideology that created the movement, and survive under varying conditions is effective. Only the complete extinction of the movement's primary goal constitutes failure. Moderate, but stable survival, is a success as well, differing in scale, not kind.

THE SOCIAL MOVEMENT
REVISITED

Margaret Mead coined the phrase, "evolutionary cluster" to express the idea that small cohorts of individuals can change the critical path of a society (Mead 1964: 145; 266). These clusters promote change by influencing the lives of individuals, the groups in the social movement, and the value "repertoire" of the society.

In a complex, goal-directed system, the system is quickly transformed by a well-known principle. After a short time, the primary goals of the system are usurped by maintenance goals. These may become more important to the system than the original aims, even contradicting the original goal (Gall 1975: 23). Translated into mundane terms, this means that no matter how lofty the original aim, the details of implementing this goal rapidly become paramount. For example, in a hospital, the primary task of medical treatment must compete with the monumental effort to stay organized, to carefully document events, and of course to keep tabs on the mountain of costs and purchases. In a social movement, the original catalytic analysis is undermined by the constructive analyses that actually direct the organization and implementation of the original goal. The primary goal, the implementation of Aquarian values, can be modified and even subordinated to the needs of the individuals in the small cells and networks.

Decisions about leadership, organization, and specific therapeutic content shape the movement's goals. Decisions to practice publicly or privately are crucial, as are the degree to which "spiritual" assumptions figure in the movement.

Each ideological stance has implications for social organization. Figure 5.4 represents the different shifts in organization that are linked with these decisions. Ultimately, the social movement can possess egalitarian, charismatically centered, and institutional organizations. Mature social movements may include stable populations of egalitarian cohorts. They will not have the obvious impact of a hierarchical structure, but they will survive.

Social movements on the scale of holistic health are subsystems of larger cultural drifts. Such macromovements are called general social movements (Blumer 1969: 9). They characteristically present more abstract, ideological, vague goals. Their leadership is indirect, attempting to steer and not govern the direction of the movement. The Aquarian conspiracy is a magnificent example. Within the ideological parameters of the general social movement, however, specific movements arise with direct behavioral goals (Blumer 1969: 11). Under the rubric of the human potential movement, Reichian consciousness, Esalen's experiments, Zen Buddhism, and Yoga proliferated (Mattson 1977: 36). Holistic health is a favored offspring of the Aquarian movement.

FIGURE 5.4 CYBERNETIC NETWORKS IN A SOCIAL MOVEMENT

PRIMARY GOAL: Changing the ideology of the culture
—changing the lives of the individuals that participate in the movement
—changing the attitudes and policies of other aspects of that culture.

SECONDARY GOALS: Develop practices that implement the Primary Goal and create networks to facilitate practice and survival.

EGALITARIAN:
Decentralized
segmented cells,
united by ideology
EXAMPLE:
Peer networks of
holistic health
practitioners,
workshops

AUTHORITARIAN
CHARISMATIC LEADERSHIP:
Leaders retain great
authority within cell
Leaders also contribute
to overall ideology of
movement
Leaders inhibit
comprehensive
institutionalization
EXAMPLE:
Theurgic organizations,
Religious "covenant"
Residential communities

INSTITUTIONAL/
HIERARCHICAL STRUCTURE:
Maximum number
of component cells fit
into organizational
framework

FIGURE 5.4 *(continued)*

	EXAMPLE:
	Professional Associations (American Holistic Medical Association, American Chiropractic Association, International Chiropractic Association, Institute for Structural Integration, i.e., Rolfers, etc.) and Churches (Emissaries of Divine Light, Unity, Church of Religious Science, etc.)

ORGANIZATIONAL INTERACTION
All three organizational types are always present and interact in personal
    networks
Membership between groups is fluid
Leadership is fluid
Ideology binds the diverse elements together
Egalitarian structure is especially difficult to eliminate

In a social movement four levels of organization are affected: the individual, the group/cell, the network, and the community at large. These are of course, nested, not mutually exclusive categories. As I review the maturation process of a social movement, it will become evident that the individual level is more important at one phase of the movement, the group in another, and so forth. As critical crossroads are reached within the movement, some practitioners will opt to stay with the stage emphasizing the individual, for that is why they joined.

Initially, in the formation of a social movement, there must be at least two preceeding factors. The first prerequisite is a dissonance, a conflict of values felt by a number of people, establishing a need for change. Second, a body of knowledge is required from which potential answers can be synthesized. Holistic health, as you saw in chapter 3, possesses a body of knowledge, from which any number of analyses can spring. Chapter 4 presented the bewildering array of historical sources that combined to create holistic health.

Once the concept of a steady state golden age is abandoned, cognitive dissonance is easy to postulate. Perfect ideological attunement to the society is inconceivable, particularly in times of rapid change. In this case, the last score of years has brought an upwelling spring of discontent. Old social structures eroded into compact, highly mobile, nucleated, urban families. American individualism took on a new meaning as isolation from kith and kin became a lifestyle. "Whole" and "holy" were ideas perceived as increasingly distant from mundane existence. In Polarity Gestalt awareness, familial alienation was literally a constant topic. In Mattson's study of holistic healers in the Bay Area, and my own experience, the overwhelming majority of practitioners were religious defectors, apostates, drawn to the values of holistic health to fill a perceived void (1977: 36). Joyce, my friend and a prime informant put it this way:

> I cry at particular things. I cry at the truth. When I
> really . . . see the truth in this world, I cry at it. It's
> like there's not enough of it. I used to think that I'm
> crying at the beauty of it. Hell no, I don't think so. I'm
> crying at the sadness of something within me. I'm sad
> that there's not more of it. Or I'm sad that it is not true
> for me . . .

From the point of view of the social movement, this discontent set the stage for ideological experimentation.

At the same time, insurance and an astonishing availability of health care transformed the American consciousness of health. The orthodox medical profession had reached an unparalleled position of power. Not everyone was content to worship at that altar. Just as a shaman with particularly strong spells is the source of both awe and distrust, the social distance of the physician inhibited complete trust (Foster and Anderson 1978: 114). Disease was becoming a scientifically esoteric entity and health its vague antithesis. This was a disturbing trend for some people. As one practitioner put it, "Modern medicine is the legacy of war and the drug industry. The miracle of modern medicine is that it is still around."

This sentiment is not unique to American culture. Otsuka's study of the revival of kanpo, traditional Chinese medicine in Japan, reveals patients' discontent with cosmopolitan medicine. Concerns about side

effects, overspecialization, social distance, and disregard of the patient as a person are contrasted with "holistic" kanpo tradition (1976:
322). This dissonance is the backdrop, not the shaping force in the
movement. The direction comes from creative solutions, synthesized
from the historical information.

In the midst of this discontent, a social movement must rally around
an individual or a small collection of persons. The analysts offer solutions to the original dissonance (Platt 1975: 267; Mead 1964: 152, 265–
67). This catalytic analysis contains the social criticism and the solution. Yet it does not cause the movement, it only permits the movement
to occur. At this point the movement can only continue if the catalytic
analysis is brought to public awareness through a variety of means—
media, literature, or rumour. Although the social structure is similar to
the "saint cults" that surround initial charismatic leadership (Blumer
1969: 18), in holistic health the leaders, the catalytic analysts, are primarily important as symbols of their ideas. For example, Reich's person is not beatified but the Reichian idea of self-responsibility is a critical rallying point for his ideological descendents.

The catalytic analysts engineer the turnarounds in values characteristic of an effective social movement. The analysts influence the kind
of social organization that occurs in the subsystems in the network.
Some favor strong organization and so teach their students. Others are
primarily ideologues or even mystagogues and may even impede
institutionalization.

The range of movement leadership in the form of spokesmen and
women is impressive. Figure 5.1 gives a brief overview of catalytic analysts in the last 150 years. Major progenitors of ideology and new practices were followed by succeeding generations of "constructive analysts", who created the social, not the conceptual, framework. Some
may have been "designated charismatic heirs" in the Weberian sense
(Weber 1868: 55), chosen by the original leader or the elite followers.
More often, students transform the original analysis, purifying it ideologically or making it more amenable to synthesis and institutional organization (Figure 5.2 provides a sample of constructive analysts). The
split in Polarity between the satvik practitioners based on Pannetier
and the rigorous purification of the practitioners of the Northwest
Coast is such a case.

The catalysts also direct the "flavor" of the implementation of the primary goals. It has long been noted that within each synthetic re-vitalization movement are "nativistic, millenarian, messianic, and re-vivalistic elements (Wallace 1956: 267). Within all the parameters of a given catalytic analysis, some features harken back to the glorious past, some create new options, and others employ "foreign" elements. Each cell emphasizes a particular element, creating its own flavor.

Aspects of the holistic health movement are nativistic—harkening back to a nobler age. Nature is now good but was better. The ancestors were healthier. One overzealous informant expressed the idea that ancient man was never sick! This has been echoed by other natural hygienists (Roth 1976: 113). Milder variations of these beliefs were widespread, especially in herbology, cleansing, or vegetarian dietary regimes. They all praise the virtues of an older age and use the overall spiritual and physical degradation of the modern environment as justification for rigid and constant purification.

Jin Shin Do illustrates the complexities of nativism. The therapy is only one component of the holistic health movement as a whole. Its practitioners can range from lay massage therapists, "professional" acupressurists, to highly organized and licensed acupuncturists. The philosophy is based on esoteric knowledge within the classic and folk East Asian medical system. The idea that the ancients had a superior understanding of ch'i flow and balance is implicit in the conversations of modern practitioners. The fact that this nativism is not ancestral to Europeans is almost a moot point. Nativism is blurred; it may be generically tribal, not linked to a particular past, but a mythic historical image. However, explanations involving endorphins, endrocrinology, the new physics, and the scientific study of "energy" are invoked to validate the ancient ways. In addition, the element of importation is ambiguous. Clearly, Jin Shin Do is not native to European or American shores. Yet by the time novices are exposed to this aspect of Chinese medicine, it does not seem alien. The ideas are so familiar—elan vital, energy manipulation, and the use of the hands as healing channels. The major center of the movement is in Santa Monica, not Seoul, after all.

Other components of holistic health are clearly new applications of modern American culture. The application of nutritional chemistry in herbs and dietary analysis, relativistic physics, and endocrinology are novel syntheses of ancient traditions and science. Innovative psychology is the most obviously creative in its psychic/rationalist syntheses

using combinations of behaviorism (biofeedback) and experiential
growth (Gestalt). Epistemological syntheses are more difficult. To
combine rationalist science and Aquarian values requires strengthen-
ing the assumption that physical reality is a mirror of the greater spiritual realm. For instance, endocrinological changes could be seen as
the gross physical mechanism for the more subtle energetic prime
movers. But rationalist explanations become strained when applied to
esoteric phenomena. Generalization is not consistent with the idea of
the unique individual. Anecdote is the only description suitable to a
unique being. The concept of macro-microcosm promotes the idea
that everything reflects all else, suggesting analogy. Analogy and anecdote logically become the most powerful scientific expressions in empirical medicine.

Importation is vital to the holistic health movement. Even more
than the European, East Asian and Ayurvedic medicine have more
clearly remained within the confines of a naturalistic medical tradition.
The introduction of Asian medical material and techniques has been
secondary to the revival of the ideas and basic assumptions listed in
chapter 2. Vital force is not just an old European esoteric or quack
idea, it is ch'i, *ki,* and prana. The ideas of Hippocratic medicine and
the esoteric tradition were reinforced by the parallel practice in two of
"the most civilized" parts of the world, India and China.

Once a catalytic analyst has identified a source of discontent and
provided a possible solution, crisis must occur to confirm the analysis.
It may be a crisis on the global scale, although a personal or familial
crisis may also promote commitment. In an examination of holistic
health practitioners in the Bay Area, Mattson noted a pattern of recruitment that paralleled my own observations. She perceived that illness
of self or family and resolution of familial/personal crises, coupled
with help from a particular therapy or philosophy cemented the commitment (1977; 40; 1982: 108–12).

Individuals already exposed to the catalytic analysis and motivated
by the pain of the crisis may form groups. These groups vary widely in
social organization—from loosely affiliated individual practitioners,
such as massage therapists and herbalists, to state level organizations of chiropractors and acupuncturists. Some may touch on well-
established organizations. The Y.M.C.A. and the Unitarian church do
not exist solely to promote holistic health, but they provide a useful

structure for recruitment and education. For example, the Paraiso Y.M.C.A. offers classes in shiatzu and Swedish massage, as well as advocating "clean living" and self-responsibility. Other groups, tightly knit, exist primarily to provide strong centers for education and practice. The Polarity Alive Fellowship is a prime illustration of a formal residential community. Several such centers are scattered over the West Coast. The one in Paraiso, now established elsewhere, offered a number of classes, workshops, and opportunities for individual therapy.

The groups share a "macro-ideology," a core of primary goals and values. In holistic health, this includes the assumptions and goals stated in chapter 2. The ideologically linked groups enter a period of expansion and recruitment, focusing on educating and reaching out to the community. This process involves the clarification of fine distinctions between groups, resulting in the appearance of schisms. The Reichians become the pure Reichians and the Neo-Reichians. Neo-Reichians may follow Charles Kelley and the Radix school, a "growth psychology" reworking of Reich's model. Neo-Reichians also include the disciples of Alexander Lowen, the creator of bioenergetics. Likewise, they may follow the seminal work of Ida Rolf, a student of Reich. Founder of Structural Integration (Rolfing), she, in turn, influenced Teresa Phrimmer, teacher of Marge Kapsos, who developed another philosophy and technique of deep muscle release. Rolf also taught Judith Aston, who combined the goals of postural change with movement therapy and created Aston Patterning.

Segmentation thus established, it is wise to begin looking at intergroup linkages and the interaction of each cell with the community. Segmentary organization in a social movement has been carefully examined by Luther Gerlach and Virginia Hine. They noted that these groups tend to be decentralized in their decision making and segmented into interacting networks (Gerlach and Hine 1973: 34–35). They are linked by ideology, a masterplan for interpreting experience (1973: 174–75).

In egalitarian organizations Gerlach and Hine found a series of leaders, guiding seemingly divergent groups, instead of strong charismatic leaders. (Gerlach and Hine 1981: 77–87). Some of the leaders were hierarchical, but most were *primus inter pares,* first among equals, comparable to ranked chiefs in a global village model (Hine 1977: 20).

They found this structure in the populations they studied, the Black Power movement, and the Pentecostal revival. They also reevaluated millennial movements, such as the Melanesian cargo cult, noting the presence of their organizational construct (Gerlach and Hine 1981: 38). In addition, Gerlach (1980) investigated the ecological movement and Hine (1980) focused on California's new age communities.

Hine was particularly interested in the way her organizational construct was reinforced by the Aquarians with a conscious focus on mutually created rituals, consisting of meaningful symbols, such as light, that bind the group into a whole and accent positive emotions (1980: 11; and personal communciation). Ferguson (1980: 217, 262) and Mattson (1982: 134) have specifically noticed the applicability of this kind of social organization in holistic health.

Recall some of the organizational features of Paraiso. The locale contains supportive citizens, catering to New Age commercial and educational needs. Health food stores, alternative public clinics, holistic health oriented institutes, workshops, and lectures are an integrated part of community. There are clients who go regularly or sporadically to holistic health practitioners. Novices are drawn from these supporting networks, and clients come from various places. These people learn the values and practices from an unceasing series of workshops and apprenticeships or from formal alternative healing academies. They may then join the majority of practitioners who prefer to practice in small, private networks, with or without official licensing, or they may choose to practice publicly. More than two-thirds of the public practitioners are teachers and group leaders. Group leaders and members alike drift in and out of the community casually. Group membership centers around teachers of the same technique, philosophy, or neighborhood. Rarely are there formal hierarchical distinctions. Leaders are also comrades, first among equals (see Gerlach and Hine 1981: 34–35; 1980: 77; Hine 1977: 21). Membership of individual cliques overlap, and status in one group may not follow a practitioner into another.

Networks develop in cultural, as well as geographic territories, with divisions over interpretations (Gerlach 1980: 77). Rapid communication is vital to maintaining network cohesion. Membership flows between networks but group identity is still distinct (1973: 164–65). This factionalism increases the potential for recruitment and makes the movement more difficult to oppose (Gerlach and Hine 1981: 66–77; Hine 1977: 19). Factionalism develops on the basis of ideology, personal or geographic cleavages, or competition for followers (Gerlach and Hine 1981: 42).

In the holistic health community novices and practitioners alike sometimes declare allegiance to a faction, becoming skeptics or supporters of a particular transformational mechanism, often playing out past schisms in the occult community during the last century. In Paraiso, a debate developed over the merits of a Sikh synthesis or Rosicrucian-based meditation. Primarily a conflict between two psychic healers, the schism affected at least fifty novices and practitioners. Each healer and his/her primary disciples castigated the merits of the opponent's spirit guides and ability to help his or her disciple to metaphysically evolve and usher in the New Age. Each found the other dogmatic. Personality, follower autonomy, and individual belief all played a part in this factionalism.

Intergroup differences are solidified. New constructive analyses are continually being made, as you saw in the Reich-Rolf-Aston-Kapsos example. Some constructive analyses refine the differences between groups, other merge them. Some focus on an ideology that precludes strong organization, others create dogma and strict living rules. Some groups pragmatically choose the loss of a fragment of the original ideology in favor of survival. Others choose demise over the loss of fundamentalism. The schism within Polarity demonstrates this principle. One faction has taken the basic principles and has transformed them into a technique, which can be used with any Aquarian philosophy. The other has taken the same ideas of Randolph Stone and made them firm guidelines for a total life-style. In Paraiso, the latter school was particularly concerned with the inability of Paraiseños to fathom innate gender differences. The stubborn citizenry was unwilling to admit that women were innately passive and men natural decision makers. It became such a critical position that, over time, the number of workshops given on this issue increased. At the same time, attendance dropped. The message was not what the Paraiseños wanted to hear. The group's position became tenuous, demonstrating that the ideological stance had professional consequences.

The force for schism is great. Underneath the differences, is there a common vision of "what is wrong and why, and how life ought to be organized?" (Meeks 1983: 173). Such questions evoke the "millennial myth." I propose that such imagery exists in the Aquarian movement, however varied the specific details.

IDEOLOGY AND GOALS

The influence of "spiritual" forces on social transformation is an area of vague general agreement, yet specific details vary. Some practitioners are oriented to a non-materialist, almost generic spiritual goal. Others concentrate on specific occult traditions. These debates emerged in the EFR interviews and are borne out by participant-observation.

The future is the fixation of a social movement. The past is gone, the present imperfect, and only the future contains the hope of a promised life. Individual practitioners' scenarios of futures have two expectations. They anticipate political and economic upheaval. In addition, they foresee a spiritual transformation of human nature. Like other theurgic millennial movements, particularly the "Free Spirit" heresy in the late Middle Ages, they hope to gain angelic or divine attributes, achieving unity and identity with pure spirit (Cohn 1970: 148–86). Voluntary simplicity, esoteric Gnostic "right thought," and protest of existing spiritual authority were features of this medieval movement (Cohn 1962: 35). They are applicable to the holistic health movement as well.

Optimistic global scenarios vary from one practitioner to another yet generally anticipate a fundamental future change in human consciousness. At least, people will be more compassionate, aware of spiritual phenomenon, and appreciative of the holiness of mankind and the planet, goals derived from humanistic psychology. Wilhelm Reich, the "father of holistic health," openly advocated transformational social change. By releasing the sexual, emotional, and cognitive blocks trapping the body, a person could be freed to be creative and sensitive to life energy (Hoffman and Mann 1980: 206–43). Reich worked for an age in which mankind would be liberated and therefore truly rational. He believed this would be a novel event in human history, once saying "human culture does not even exist yet" (1980: 205). Reich worked on children, hoping that some would survive the chaos he saw as the inevitable result of modern society.

Others actively anticipate a semi-divine stage in which the chosen will be psychically powerful and ecologically wise. This is only an intermediate point, since at this stage it is impossible to envision true divinity. An example of this scenario has been published in a science fiction novel written by Thea Alexander (1976), *2150 A.D.* Although fiction, it is used as a set of instructions. The author teaches workshops and sells books in Arizona to spread her world view. The book is widely read in Holistic/New Age circles. It is the saga of sub-macro man, an evolutionary step above micro man. Micro-man is selfish, unaware of cosmic unity and karma—the subtle set of lessons of past mistakes, repeated until learned. The story revolves around Jon and Karl. In his dreams, Jon goes to 2150 and the nearly utopian macro society. He returns to graduate school when awake. In the macro society he learns that macro consciousness began in the 1970s and 1980s. After fierce political and environmental convulsions macro society had survived, guided by enlightened network leaders and computers.

Social collapse, and the battle for domination are vital to these worst case scenarios. The contemporary social elite (including occasionally medical physicians) may fill the rival role, and there may be a spiritual component to the contest.

In the pessimistic scenario the massive upheavals are the result of actions by adepts who manipulate governments, money, and consumer taste to further their own ambitions. Occult traditions may supply the content of these beliefs. One example involves stories of the Illuminati, based on several fiction and nonfiction books by Robert Shea and Robert Anton Wilson (for a self-analytical explanation of the novels see Wilson 1978). They developed the novels, based on the historic "materialist," republican secret society nested in the Freemasons (Crow 1968: 279–80). The Illuminati are alternately the antagonists or the protagonists. They are conceptually linked with international banking, the Roman Catholic Church (for or against), visitors from Sirius, Aleister Crowley, and Timothy Leary. The significant feature of this scenario is that it emphasizes the esoteric nature of global conflict. Portraying political conflict as a red herring, the novels of the Illuminati point to a struggle of those with special knowledge.

Another tradition involves a reincarnation of the struggle between the indulgent, self-gratifying inhabitants of Mu and the intellectual Atlanteans, doomed to relive until they can learn compassion and brotherly love (Bailey 1980). This signifies the importance of karma. In the holistic health community this refers to understanding spiritual and

stic healers and a belief that the power elite have failed. Disasters portrayed by the media heighten this feeling (Barkun 1974: 61).

Recall that some informants, namely leaders in the holistic health community, have a unified vision of best, worst, and probable scenarios. They also have more faith, if you will, that their millennial mechanisms will be the agents of change. Although the scenarios are often painful, the promise of the new age eases the anxiety.

Aquarian spirituality is the unifying vision of the millennial promise. Humanity would be "embedded in nature," decentralized, interdependent but autonomous (Ferguson 1980: 29). The Aquarian values form a template for the future, one transformed by spiritual and terrestrial reformation.

INSTITUTIONS AND HERESIES: A COMPARATIVE EXAMPLE FROM EARLY CHRISTIANITY

The people that pursue millennial promises form social groups. However, the critical question revolves around the nature of those groups. Do they inevitably become institutions, sealing the promises into dogma? In pursuing the literature on social movements, I was struck by two common assumptions. First, it is taken for granted that Weberian institutionalization is the proper destiny of a social movement. A "successful" movement becomes an established formal organization. Second, it was assumed that institutions implemented their primary goals—the promises that created the original social movement.

There is an alternative to these assumptions. In addition to institutionalization, egalitarian, decentralized groups may keep a movement intact. Moreover, institutionalization may actually subvert the goals of the movement. The survival of the hierarchy may become more important than the survival of the original movement's message. The history of early Christianity provides some crosscultural, historical evidence for the survival of heresy, along with the well known formal institution. The first few centuries of Christianity have better documentation than any other comparable movement (Meeks 1983: 1). It is a movement steeped in history. Antecedents of Christianity, the forces for schism, and the formation of the Church orthodoxy have fascinated social historians. Ethnicity, political affiliation, class/status ambiguity, and even theology created factions in the first three centuries of the early Christian movement. Cox (1978) suggests that comparing the fertile first centuries of Christianity with modern movements might shed light on both. Studying the early Christian movement reveals processes relevant to the survival of holistic health and the Aquarian conspiracy.

Several critical questions are involved in this comparison. First, was the social structure of early Christianity broad enough to allow for the creation of many alternatives? Second, was the institutionalization itself a point of controversy in the movement? Third, did the alternatives survive the institutionalization of the movement?

Early Christianity demonstrates many of the themes of the cycle of a social movement—cultural dissonance, the use of pre-existing networks for recruitment, and constructive analyses by later members. The social networks that formed the early movement were varied, linked primarily by ideology, not common background.

During the first century after the death of Christianity's messiah, the direction of the movement was open to interpretation. The alliance of James with Judaic culture and Paul with the Gentiles was a critical point. The Roman Empire at that time provided a milieu for travel and trade not seen again until the nineteenth century (Meeks 1983: 17). The conversion of Paul, with his Hellenistic, urban tradesmen affiliations broadened the social base (Meeks 1983: 17–26, 109). Paul was in a unique position to be a culture broker for Hellenistic Jews and the "God-fearing." The latter were the basis for many networks in early Christianity. Drawn to Judaism, but reluctant to commit themselves through adult circumcision, they provided a pool of hosts and allies for Paul and his followers. The use of preexisting networks to broaden a social movement is a powerful tool (Gerlach and Hine 1981: 97).

The early Christians, it now appears, were often tradesmen and bourgeoisie in a society that had not yet created a niche for the middle class. A wealthy slave may not have been materially deprived, but he was still a slave. A landowner may have benefited from Roman rule but felt ethical qualms. There were no simple class breakdowns.

Meeks suggests that the ambiguity itself was a more compelling context for early Christianity than disaffection of the marginal (1983: 10–15). His idea is a logical position, paralleling other social movements including holistic health. Moreover, a struggle of the rural and urban poor would not have created the networks that extended over Roman Asia.

The early Empire in Asia and Africa was a fount of opportunity—
new possibilities were created from eroding social contraints. Families
were "breaking down" (Dodds 1965: 115) and familial traditions were
no longer absolute bonds with the past. It became more common for
members of a family to change classes and to have different religions
(Meeks 1983: 30–31). This had obvious implications for recruitment. It
was easier to recruit three people out of twenty, than all twenty. Although this led to the use of Christianity as a scapegoat for familial
discord, it created more cells in the network.

Early Christianity was rife with diversity. Interpretations developed
out of the ideological potpourri and geographically dispersed networks. Choices—*hairesis* (the root word of heresies)—abounded.
The ancient physician/philosopher Celsus wrote that the new religion
was split into many warring sects, united only by the name "Christian"
(Dodds 1965: 103).

The issue every social movement must confront is authority and organization. In early Christianity, this was hotly debated and became a
point of divergence. Although the early bishopry was roughly egalitarian within its own ranks, there was agreement among the orthodox that
there should be ranks. The powerful Novations, the "puritans" of the
early church, asserted that "no one could have God for his Father, who
has not the Church for his Mother" (Bruce 1978: 213). Some heresies
denied this. Although the Valentinian Gnostics of the fourth century
vainly tried to reconcile the egalitarian Gnostics and the developing
hierarchy, most of the Gnostics persisted in rampant individualism.
Their trinity embraced the female principle, and their rotating clergy
included women (Pagels 1981: 59–70). Abrogating the omnipotence of
the God of Abraham (1981: 40–41), the literal resurrection of the body
(1981: 7–9), and even the corporeal existence of Jesus (1981: 121–22)
minimized the innate authority of the orthodoxy. Indeed, the Gnostics
referred to the new hierarchy as "waterless canals" (Pagels 1981: 29).
The Gnostic fixation with individual theurgy, spiritual evolution, and
intuitive understanding was offensive to the orthodoxy. The idea of individual, multiple truths was not compatable with routinization of
charismatic leadership.

Some individuals chose the decentralized course, precisely because it was neither institutionalized nor allied with fixed authority. For
example, the Donatists of the fourth and fifth centuries did not want to
become friends with the empire and actively sought martyrdom (Frend

1976: 20). Such reactions were consistent for those portions of the social movement that rebelled against the status quo.

During, and even after, the creation of the Catholic Church and its
incorporation into the Roman Empire, the religious movement was not
a monolithic entity. The Gnostic collection of heresies provided a good
example the diversity in early Christianity.

Gnosticism was partially a response to the Judaic nature of Christianity. The "dialogue with paganism" began early as followers of Paul
and Apollos in Corinth, and later Marcion, converted gentiles and absorbed Hellenistic philosophy. The position of Marcion in A.D. 150 was
the most extreme. His rhetoric suggested that with the transformative
acts of Jesus, none of the more archaic forms of Judaism were necessary. Judaic ideas and writings "contaminated" the pure form of Christianity. To this end, Marcion wrote a revised Gospel for the New Testa-
ment. In it, there were two gods—the greater god and the inferior
Jewish one (Bruce 1978: 228, 249–50).

The theological debate on the nature of the Christian god was continued by the Gnostics. They referred to the Jewish god as Samael, god
of the blind. They postulated that the Judaic god governed the sphere
of the mundane, unaware of his own limitations until the greater Father
and Mother (Wisdom) informed him. This had an impact on the development of the church, the hierarchical organization. Divine omnipotence was the theoretical foundation of church authority. By denying
the omnipotence of the God of Abraham, the Gnostics rejected the authority of the developing clergy. Platonism—the emphasis on the spiritual plane of the ideal—took root in alternative cells in Christianity.
The Valentinian Gnostics and the theologian Origen (active A.D. 203–
248) wove sophisticated, Hellenistic philosophical arguments supporting their Christianity. The Greco-Roman pagans courted these synthesists, hoping to incorporate them into intellectual polytheism (Dodds
1965: 107). The Valentinians resisted, but this probably did not endear
them to the purists. As the church father Tertullian expounded, "Away
with all attempts to produce a mixed Christianity" (Pagels 1981: 137).

Tertullian's wish was not entirely fulfilled. The legalization and
codification of Christianity in the fourth century made diversity more
difficult. Despite the discourse concerning the "demise" of heresies,
mystical and esoteric traditions continued, echoing heretical notions.
This does not mean that later Christian mystics were part of a conspiracy to keep gnosticism alive, but simply that in a decentralized, egali-

tarian structure, ideas are hard to crush. This is the advantage of such structure (Gerlach and Hine 1981: 66–77). A system with many scattered leaders is difficult to eliminate. In this case, the dominance of the orthodox Roman Catholic church did not make it the only representative of the Christian doctrine. Diversity survived.

Neonatal Christianity highlights some of the principles of a social movement discussed in this chapter. It illustrates the broad, diverse social networks that are vital in establishing a social movement. Christianity possessed varied social organizations—elaborate hierarchical institutions and decentralized egalitarian structures. The latter structure is relevant in discussing the success and survival of the diversity in a movement. This choice was a point of divergence in the tradition of early Christianity. It produced a sudden shift (catastrophe) that reshaped the later traditions. Because some elements in Christianity were not highly organized, they managed to persist in spite of opposition.

This persistence suggests that a social movement might include two consequences—institutionalization and decentralized survival. The way in which this choice affects the holistic health movement is the focus of chapter 7. The role of the individual in a decentralized organization is the subject of chapter 6.

BECOMING A HEALER

Learning is finding out what you already know. Doing is demonstrating that you know it. Teaching is reminding others that they know just as well as you. You are all learners, doers, teachers. (Illusions, Bach: 1984: 58)

The holistic health movement stands between a long tradition of empirical healing and a millennial hope and vision for the future. At the same time this social movement is the translator of the hopes of the individual practitioner. The goals and values of the social movement provide a learning template for the individual and provide a social group in which learning occurs. Fully socialized members of the holistic health movement can teach other potential practitioners, clients, friends, and even anthropologists. For holistic health practitioners, learning the movement's values happens simultaneously with acquiring the skills of empirical healing, becoming "shamans-in-civilization."

This chapter refers both to the processes of movement conversion and to the empirical medical education of holistic health practitioners. For example, recruitment not only involves the process of attraction and conversion to the Aquarian ideals, but also choosing a career in holistic health. This involves learning a new set of values, skills, and even a new style of cognition. The holistic health practitioner must develop the ability to perceive other subtle realities, to discern the small energy differences in the body of a client. Detecting the invisible and reinterpreting the mundane for the client requires a special state of

mentioned chiropractors and 38 percent of the holistic health practitioners in Mattson's study (1982: 108). In my key informants' life histories, first contact with holistic health did not center on a dramatic crisis or cure, but alternative care of a crisis promoted curiosity and commitment to the movement. For example, Doug, a pioneer in Paraiso's counterculture, had felt isolated and "uptight." Much to his later amusement and horror he had been an accountant. He was shy, alienated, and had suffered a lifetime of colds. He felt an urgent need to change his life. He learned massage, took sensitivity training in Los Angeles, and was then involved with a traffic accident that broke the patterns in his old life. He was Rolfed—that is, given a series of deep-tissue body work treatments. His resolve was reinforced by his improvement, and he became a practitioner and teacher. Chronic and acute illness, and especially accidents, drew the awareness of the future practitioners to their own bodies.

For Doug, being Rolfed was the first step to becoming a body-worker. Going to a chiropractor usually preceeds becoming one. Being a client, however, is not itself training. Michael Harner, in his fascinating how-to book on shamanism, *The Way of the Shaman: A Guide to Power and Healing* (1980), points out that becoming a shaman is a matter of "individual experience," based on learned methods.

Harner suggests that learning these methods from a book is an appropriate method (1980: xii). For a novice in a literate society, this is the first step. Drawn in by Theosophical texts such as Norman Cousin's *Anatomy of an Illness* (1979) or Ferguson's *The Aquarian Conspiracy* (1980), potential practitioners begin to read and consider. Books have a way of becoming the center of ad hoc study groups. Established practitioners come into this fertile ground and give workshops, and the workshops become organized programs. Some individuals then seek apprenticeships. One informant suggested that the only real way to learn homeopathy was to study under a master, learning case by case.

Legally, socially, and structurally, however, the most attractive method in American society is the specialized school/clinic. This is a society where even a gardener can go to a community college or a trade school and learn his trade. Holistic health is based on the idea of healing as an empirical craft. Where better to learn a skill than a craft center? International guides such as *Wholistic Dimensions in Healing: A Resource Guide* (Kaslof 1978) have been compiled to help locate the center corresponding to an area of interest: childbirth, integrative medical systems, nutrition and herbs, metaphysical groups, bodywork, and new age psychology. Local guides are produced at the community level, cooperative efforts designed to make potential healers and clients aware of their nearby resources. Drawn to a particular approach, often through personal experience, a client then chooses to learn that method as a practitioner. Doug, for example, having experienced the benefits of Rolfing, as well as Esalen massage and sensitivity awareness, went to an institute that taught techniques similar to Rolfing, but combined other interests as well. Within that academy, and the ones I attended, values, techniques, and new ways of thinking are learned by a band of novitiates.

LEARNERS, DOERS, TEACHERS

In a loft office/school in central Paraiso, novice healers gathered to learn their new craft. Practitioners also used the center as a meeting place to integrate new ideas into their existing practices. For its impact on the holistic health community the surroundings were homey and unpretentious. The reception area—more like a principal's than a doctor's office—was distinguished by the presence of herbs, specialty books, and nearby photographs of happy teachers and graduates. The class area was decorated with anatomy charts, punctuated by posters of East Asian meridians. Massage tables doubled as practice surfaces and as desks—although most lectures ended up with students taking notes while sitting cross-legged on the floor. Adjoining was a kitchen/patio where students and instructors collected at the break for herb tea and an occasional fruit feast. Down the hall the shower/dressing room stood across from Patrick's office—part library and part clinic. Occasionally interrupted by the discordant tones of a neighboring disco, this center for holistic health practice seemed like an island of academic intensity, coupled with spirituality and relaxation.

In this context, the novices had to learn the values of the social movement and the skills of holistic health practitioners. Group reinforcement was essential to both of those tasks. Armed with pasts littered with esoteric and medical literature, workshops, and experiences as clients, each member of the group was a student and a teacher. Learning was done by practicing on each other, and as many hours were spent on the table as over it. Every day, perhaps several time that day, a new body, with unique aches, demands, and expertise was placed before the novice. Even the instructors were not exempt from the efforts of the trainees. Techniques were learned with the use of handbooks, combining lofty ideals with how-to illustrations. Students gathered around a demonstration of a particular technique, narrated by the group leader and punctuated with comments from the body on the table. Technical skills could only be gained through actual experience, acting as trainee practitioner and client to another novice. They learned the explicit teaching of skills and techniques, and also the nuances of appropriate interpersonal behavior that incorporate the ideas and values of the Aquarian experience.

The novices I worked beside formed small groups, learning to strengthen their own identity as a peer group and as part of a professionalizing ideological network. The healers had to learn to share a new "moral code," a set of assumptions about the nature of health in cosmic perspective. They tested each new behavior to see if it was appropriate and consistent with their code. Although the assumptions behind the code were set forth in chapter 1 their repetition here casts them in a new light.

Each novice is taught to sense the internal feeling of the life force, the tingling, streaming, shivering energy that makes people qualitatively different from rocks. They are taught that illness stems from blocking this force, and that humans are more than mere material entities, they are material shadows of life energy. As energy beings, the practitioners are trained to use their energy to influence others. The techniques and intentions vary but the theme remains constant. The potential healers are shown how facial features, irises, postures, dreams, images, and words all reflect a larger reality about the client—and themselves. They are constantly reminded not to work from an ideal, but with an individual unique person who is dynamic and changing. The new practitioners should monitor each step of the therapy, and change when change is required. They are taught to reflect on their own lives, just as their clients are taught to reflect on the nature of illness as a lesson. Why is this cold, muscle spasm, or tumor happening at this time? What is to be learned? Finally, after the fashion of the Neoplatonists, they learn to recognize different levels of existence, physical, emotional, cognitive, and spiritual. The spheres are linked and the most powerful is spirit. Practitioners are, therefore, taught to recognize undifferentiated holiness, the spirit, and to function in an alternative reality of imagination and symbol. Within this reality, spirit forces can be balanced and harmony restored. Satvik balancing touches are used to "feel" the energy flow back and forth, until the two sides of the body, or the two "strange flow" points, or the two areas of tension are relaxed, restored, and flowing freely.

This approach aims directly at restoring empathy and spirituality into the client/healer relationship. This is the mode of the modern holistic healer reflecting the values of the New Age. This differs markedly from sociological studies of the socialization of cosmopolitan medical doctors (Zabarenko and Zabarenko 1978: 39–40). During training, just as they are developing empathy, medical students are exposed to traumatic encounters with cadavers and a host of impersonal information. This activity tends to negatively reinforce patient/doctor empathy and becomes a critical issue in the development of professional roles and the coexistence of the two traditions, to be explored in chapter 7.

The instruction of empathy is a vital part of holistic healer education. How does an individual learn to be a holistic healer?" I had automatically hypothesized that their behavior was reinforced by others in the group. To a certain extent this is true but insufficient. In training and practice, the immediate and rewarding primary reinforcements are available: hugs, grins, caresses, and sweet words. However, simple reinforcement schemes have limitations in understanding social movements (see Cantril 1963: 55–56). How do people know when to reinforce each other, particularly in the setting of the novitiate?

The educational setting is the key. Workshops and "craft schools" provide a special learning situation. Learning is a constant, dynamic process, shaped by subtle factors in the environment. Successful self-change—the key to movement conversion and professional rites of passage—must be preceeded by self-knowledge, goal clarification, planning, new information, and modification of ones mental plan (Tharp and Watson 1977: 3–12). How is this accomplished?

Answering that question demands consideration of "high level reinforcement." Human beings watch their environments carefully and produce models. The fields of cognitive psychology, systems theory, and artificial intelligence have tentatively explored this modeling. A system cannot wait until it is reinforced by the environment, for that reinforcement may be fatally negative. A complex system must anticipate negative reinforcements and react to warnings, not the actual stimulus (Kauffman 1980: 15, 30). In artificial intelligence development this is called creating "predictive memory modules," based on internal world views. Given any new information, we integrate it. Will Z happen, if I do Y? Any creature possessing such a memory structure can hypothesize an action and receive a mental image of the results before the action is performed (Albus 1981: 137). To do this, people have to acquire new abstract information, such as the moral code of the social movement. They then have a backdrop against which to test appropriate and inappropriate behavior (see Geyer 1980: 15, 152; Mandler 1984: 66–83). Practitioners do not have to wait for the hugs in every case. Cultural beings are creatures who have imagination and the ability to anticipate circumstances and forecast the results of our actions. Experiences can be created in the imagination that have never occurred. Given a goal, these mental meanderings can become planning, projections of favorable scenarios (Albus 1981: 220–23). Abstract models of morality can be used to run a little subroutine, a mental simulation of intended behavior and expected social consequences.

This can work particularly well under three conditions that occur during the novice's training. First, the mental model must be clearly articulated. People must know the code. This is provided through literature and discussion. Second, while people are learning what is to be valued, they are constantly judging behavior against the code, daydreaming and planning, expanding the range of the code (Albus 1981: 223–24; Langfield 1979: 134). Third, a social environment devoted to those values, where all are committed to reinforcing the same values, can use simulations most effectively. The community is caught up in the new and different behavior. There is no time or energy for old patterns (Platt 1971: 6). It is no coincidence that the leaders of the learning academy in Paraiso emphasize that the initial twelve week class modules are designed to restructure the lives of the students. In this newly formed community the good opinion of peers, leaders, and eventually clients is a strong motivation to run these imaginary scenarios and constantly revise behavior and perfect the understanding of the code (Goffman 1967; 1970: 10–12; Garfinkel 1967: 35–49). We find a small working group acting with other groups to form a community. These decentralized communities form a larger network. The individuals in this network act together, though separately, to promote common beliefs and plans. These beliefs and plans are learned in a subtle fashion through group interaction, personal reflection, and choice. These choices permeate everyday life. The foods eaten, clothes worn, books read are statements about the holistic health lifestyle. They affect how a person acts by him/herself, in a group, and with a client.

These learning choices start with the individual. The moral reality defined in holistic healing requires one overwhelming attitude. A person, particularly a healer, must always be aware of the body's feelings, reactions, and needs. For example, Asian acupuncturists are encouraged, if not required, to practice on themselves long before they touch another person (Academy of Traditional Chinese Medicine 1975: 9). A holistic healer emulates this ideal.

Acupuncture point locations, various massage techniques, herbs and dietary changes are all self-administered by the novice. Echoes of Thomsonian self-help are combined with self-awareness. If a trainee were to have menstrual cramps, likely since many novices are female, this would give her an opportunity to try those new acu-points, one at the pubic symphysis and the other at Bladder meridian 1, at the glabella—a point between the eyebrows. She might also try various herbs to relieve the cramps, promote intestinal purity, and build up her overall female constitution. She might change her diet to omit salt and sugars. She might try exercises such as the polarenergetics squat or the pyramid—legs stretched akimbo, producing a gratifying pelvic pop. She might also work on her attitude. Why does she have cramps? Does she resent or fear her femaleness? Self-analysis is part of her training as a practitioner, for those are the kind of practices she might impart to a client. She should have the sensitivity to be able to identify and empathize with the feelings and complaints of the client's person. This constant attention to the status of self must be learned. It is, by necessity, a solitary activity. This must be practiced alone. It can, however, be expressed in the group.

The self-consciousness and group sharing produces a valuable learning state. I call it "holistic hypochondria." The subjective state is interpreted through the holistic paradigm. It is a beginning effort to grasp some diagnostic techniques. For example, an apprentice healer might feel pain or stiffness in the back of the neck, along the trapezius, near the temporal lobes, under the scapula near the spine or along the anterior deltoid on the upper arm. Using a Chinese paradigm, the pain points to the gall bladder meridian, a channel of energy said to govern the distribution of nutrients and balance total energy (Selinsky n.d.).

After the person has shared these discomforts with the learning

group, the initial tendency is to overwhelm the person with every con-
ceivable therapy to "cure" their colleague client. This is where the ideology of holistic health is invoked to modify action. "Curing" is an act
one does to another body, and is not consistent with dealing with the
whole person. Such action does not recognize the educational value of
the ailment, or change the behavior that led to the disharmony. Therefore, what should the student healers do for their comrade?

If you redefine the client/healer relationship to be one of mutual
education, then actions proceed differently. The healer asks questions
about lifestyle. The gall bladder meridian is associated with irritation,
frustration, and indecisiveness. What is happening in the life of that
body on the table? What is the person eating? Too much fat and not
enough vitamin A are associated with problems in this meridian (Teeguarden 1978: 34; Thie 1979: 88–89). Finally, is there another complex
of complaints and signs which imply yet another meridian such as the
lung or the spleen? Only after various interpretations have been considered, does the body get its "work." The treatments may come from
any of a wealth of techniques discussed in chapter 3. Acupressure,
dietary changes, Chinese tonic herbs, and visualizations may be used.
The work may involve Neo-Reichian breath release or Gestalt psycho-
drama. The therapy is a response to the complex of signs in that particular body and no two therapies are exactly alike.

In the holistic health academy I attended, advanced novices, those
with basic massage or health enhancement skills are encouraged to
attend a weekly "internship." This consists of supervised bodywork on
drop-in clients. These clients are often novices or practitioners themselves, desiring to be the body on the table, not over it. This provides
an opportunity for the students to meet new situations, create solutions, and compare those solutions with peers, clients, and the super-
visor. Each of these intern sessions are a preparation for professional
contacts with clients. In addition, students often work on friends and
family, forming the basis of their clientele as lay or professional
practitioners.

Working on experienced clientele is fruitful. The body on the table
is aware of internal states and how they are being affected by the novice. Verbal feedback is encouraged. The nonverbal and paralinguistic
cues, that is, thrashing, grunting, and screaming, are also effective in-
dicators of practitioner insensitivity. The experienced clients know the

rules. They can relax completely and are capable of expressing emotion freely. They know what insights they should be having. The experienced clients provide new vistas for the novice's developing internal world view.

This world view is tested when the new practitioner is exposed to uninitiated clients. The client might have little or no knowledge of the world view of holistic health. All the questions asked of the fellow healer in training sessions are restated in greater detail. Not only does the healer want to get the information necessary to understand the client's status but to educate the client about holistic health as well. The healer must explain the concept of life force and teach the client, through word and bodywork, how to recognize it. The practitioner needs to teach the person on the table that it is possible to reinterpret sensations and experiences in light of larger social and cosmic realities. The migraine can be seen anew as a lesson about the person's social interactions. The client must take some responsibility for creating and eliminating this malaise. Fostering dependency is improper for a practitioner. The idea is to "teach a hungry man to fish, not open up a fish market" (Goa 1982: 245–46). At the same time, creating a long-term "learning" relationship can pay the practitioner's rent and improve the client's self-knowledge. This fashion of therapy/education extends the range of the social movement, for yet another person can use that paradigm as a model. Articulating the tenets of the social movement in an educational or therapeutic setting exposes the beliefs to a wider audience. Using this internal world view to make behavioral choices strengthens these beliefs within the holistic healing community. Thus, a novice learns to think and act as a holistic healer. In this process the relationship between client and healer is significant.

There is wide variation in the degree of rapport advocated between practitioner and client. The poles of the continuum focus on authority and cognitive style. At one end, typified by polarity practitioners, the person over the table represents authority and knowledge. They discourage excessive empathy, pointing out that it attracts bad energy and entities. Obedience is required, otherwise, the client is not doing his "work." Threats of cutting off treatment, verbal chides, snorts, and jeers are aimed at the uncooperative client. There are few ways for the client to express psychological and physical pain. Client complaints are perceived as antagonism. Cooperation is rewarded by praise and gentleness. Polarity practitioners are trained to work with particular goals in mind, often related to Indian religious ideals, as perceived by Americans.

This contrasts with practitioners who advocate wholehearted empathy and sensitivity to the client's needs. Orthobionomy, Trager, and Jin Shin Do epitomize this approach. The therapies are deliberately nonintrusive and painless. They attempt to increase awareness of subtle energy and encourage the client to seek equilibrium. Practitioners nurture their clients. Practitioners also possess a wealth of technical knowledge, but they employ it in empathic interaction with the body on the table. The practitioner "must listen to the body at that moment," ignoring fancy techniques if they intrude on the empathy. In orthobionomy, feedback from the client is law. Complaints of pain and discomfort are to be respected. Many solutions should be presented to the client, and only she/he should choose the most appropriate.

Of course, potential clients and practitioners alike are drawn to the perspective they prefer. Practitioners can go back and forth between the authority and empathy poles, based on internal cues and the desires of the clients. Some clients will be impatient with the empathic approach, and long for visible therapy, complete with very perceptable pain. The proverb, "no gain without pain," lurks in the minds of clients and practitioners alike. I suggest that both the highly empathic state and the more assertive authoritarian state produce an awareness distantly similar to the shamanic altered state of consciousness.

THE HEALING MIND

Values, techniques, and rapport skills are learned through interpersonal feedback. The mind set of an individual healer is learned by group cues, as well as subtle psychosomatic perceptions, referred to in some peer groups as "a body buzz." The aim, as it is in shamanistic practices, is to be able to move, at will, between the ordinary state of consciousness and an altered state (Harner 1980: xiii–xvi, 48). Both are considered equally valid, with perhaps a slight bias toward the spiritual. Conversations flip casually between discussions of hairdressers, spouses, and massage oil to reincarnations, sensing auras, and chatting with one's spirit guides. Anatomical concerns are interspersed with discussions of inherited karma. This is a necessary skill.

After all, clients are going to ask questions and chat while the practitioner must be concentrating on visualizing energy. The cognitive shift is seldom dramatic when perceived from the outside. It is a purely internal, personal experience. The perceptions can be shared with the group, however, and should be in the context of the novice. Individuals who fail to "feel" the distinction are encouraged to look for perceptual cues. Feeling of heat and cold are the most easily detected. The healer Pat Taylor described the sensations experienced by southwestern healer Jewel Babb:

> During a treatment, she holds her hands out, palms toward the patient. She says a sensation of warmth starts in one of her hands, then arcs to the other, and that the energy and warmth seem to circulate in the palms. Sometimes, this energy can become so intense in her hands that she says it can cause her discomfort . . . (Taylor 1981: 25).

This warmth is the initial sensation to be felt; in energy sensitive therapies such as Jin Shin Do, this sensation mounts to produce what novices call "french fried fingers." They are then taught to tune in to more subtle differences between left and right hands and to grow sensitive to streaming sensations that have no proper English adjectives to describe them, but can be vaguely called full, empty, hollow, or sluggish. There are exercises performed to hone this skill. At one point, bodies on the table were treated with rotating novices who circle from person to person, never quite touching the person, sensing minute differences in energy quality. Each novice writes down his/her perceptions of that particular body and moves on. After every novice has worked on every body, the "charts" produced by each novice are compared. The reasons for sensing fullness in the left shoulder of Steve are discussed by all who perceived that fullness. It is an utterly empirical, sensory experience. Another training exercise involved doing a standard bodywork routine on a fellow novice while blindfolded. Tactile, and especially "energetic" sensations are the only guide. Ultimately, this skill becomes a form of divination, sensing the spiritual. Adepts at this technique do not need to ask questions of their clients, they can intuit imbalance, tension, and pain with only the lightest touch or even through off-the-body "contact."

Besides the direct attempt at sensing the etheric, novices are taught visualization routines to aid them in their foray into the invisible. Finding an "imaginary" place of power, meeting spirit guides and archetypes, and controlling the light and purity of one's own chakras are methods of manipulating the other awareness. In one such guided imagery venture, novices were led by the group leader along a specific spiritual path, asked to submerge all other thoughts and envision the leader's images using esoteric Rosicrucian symbols, to find their spirit guides. The novices were led through an image of a spinning wheel of light, through a rainbow, and up twenty-one stairs. At the top, mundane life issues were symbolically manipulated on a television screen. Seven more stairs brought the novice to meet his/her archetype child. Gifts were exchanged. Then one's energy companions/selves— personal spirit guides—introduced themselves and chatted. Powerful personal advice was given and knowledge was revealed. The guides were now known allies and could be invoked for a variety of events, including diagnostic advice. Afterward, the novice is brought back to everyday reality, having experienced the power of light/color/healing on subjective reality. Often, the thrust was not toward gaining personal power but maintaining personal defense. Frequent use of energetic perception and empathy may sully the healer's own energy. Novices are taught techniques for flushing energy through one's own body and the client's, an automatic procedure, for the healer's own safety. Shorting the energy by touching water and cognitively linking to ordinary reality are prophylactic procedures. Grounding techniques, such as visualizing roots or a golden cord to the earth, are used to help the practitioner return quickly and completely to the ordinary state of consciousness. They are imaginary visual paths back to the earth.

Holistic health practitioners seek to refine that control. Practitioners recognize a kinship to the psychotics who perceive the "other reality," but maintain that the mentally ill lack the control necessary to use that knowledge and return to commonplace reality. For the holistic health community, the lack of control and not the perception is the defining feature of psychosis. Control over creative daydreams is essential. Lack of control causes spiritual vulnerability, a state where cosmic tricksters thrive and energy goes out of balance. In the worst case, lack of control leads to psychosis or irreparable spiritual damage. Control and an altered state of perception are the basic elements of the shamanic trance (Rogers 1982; Peters and Price-Williams 1980: 398).

ALTERED STATES

Shamanic trance is not a uniform phenomenon. It ranges from light meditative trance to ecstatic dissociative trance and possession. Non-possession trance is rarely amnesic, full memory is retained (Bourguignon 1973: 12). It can be induced through reduction in motor activity, emotional hyperarousal, decreased alertness and hyperventilation, hypoxemia, dehydration, hypoglycemia, sleep deprivation, exposure to extreme temperatures, and physical pain (Jilek 1982: 226–27, 336). Neher's controlled, but to date unreplicated, study indicated that rhythm can also induce perceptual changes, such as the resistance to pain (Jilek 1982: 327–28; Price 1982: 414). Any of these may describe the client's experiences during a treatment and the novice healer is the client during his training. In this training, he/she learns to recognize the "flow of energy."

In addition, motor hyperactivity and focused and selected hyper-alertness produce altered states of awareness (Jilek 1982: 328). These conditions are common in bodywork and emotional release. Chiropractic, acupuncture, herbology, and other learned empirical skills are less overtly shamanistic. Even in "traditional" societies, such as the Bomvana of South Africa or the Kamba of Kenya, not every healer is a shaman. Herbalists, bonesetters, and midwives can practice their crafts with a minimum of spiritual inspiration (Foster and Anderson 1978: 104–8). These more earthly practices still have spiritual and energetic overtones. A salient selling point in holistic health, to clients and practitioners alike, is the momentary brush with the sublime.

The altered awareness of practitioner and practitioner-as-client is a heterogeneous affair. Perceptions range from mild meditative states to ecstatic catharsis for the clients, and perhaps practitioners, of some therapies. The meditative state was more common for the holistic. health practitioner in my experience. Kenneth Pelletier, interested in both the psychology of meditation and holistic medicine, points out that meditation may arise from either diffuse or focused attention (1977: 192–232). The key, as it is in a shamanic trance, lies in forming an internal locus of control. Successful autogenic training, a form of meditation, echoes the requirements for inducing an altered state of consciousness, but adds high motivation, cooperation of the meditator, reduction of external stimuli, and concentration on somatic stimuli as factors (Pelletier 1977: 232). Sensitive and nonaroused states come and go quickly. Visualization can be used "to mobilize the resources of both the body and the mind" (Pelletier 1977: 251). For the practitioner, concentrating on the perception of tactile, visual, and energetic cues and working with constant physical intensity for at least an hour, if not more, provide conditions that are ripe for an altered awareness. He/she is surrounded in all likelihood by recorded tapes of rhythmic music or natural sounds. The importance of the rhythm in breath and motion in body work accentuate the meditative state.

The serene, centered image of the practitioner with the relaxed client before her is not entirely representative. Holistic health is also based on a paradigm of purification, elimination, and release. Not every client is gently coaxed into self-awareness and self-healing. Some clients prefer more dramatic and rapid measures, deep muscle and tissue work, purging, intense emotional release, and catharsis. Daily coffee enemas and bodies writhing in voluntarily induced pain, struggling to rid themselves of toxins, are not serene images. It is difficult to establish the same empathic rapport in that therapeutic setting. Admittedly, this may reflect my own discomfort upon inflicting pain, but the rapport is different. Control and knowledge are more important, in this case, than close client/practitioner rapport. The emotional level is higher and the physical requirements are greater in the more tomasic therapies. Recipients of the therapies enter an altered cognitive state. Heightened sensitivity to temperature, trembling, and a profound euphoria are common reactions. I surely found it to be so. Those sensations are, in the opinion of various practitioners-as-clients, worth the pain. One polarity practitioner stated that once he had felt that way, it would be worth any effort to feel it again.

Ultimately, some practitioners link this dramatic release with sexuality. They define the energy released in these dramatic therapies as "cosmic sexual energy." The streaming, pulsating energy sought by client and practitioner is identified with Wilhelm Reich's orgone energy (Senf 1979: 110). Sexuality is the fount of life energy for Reichian, polarity, and Ayurvedic therapists alike. Reich contended that sexual potency—the ability to surrender to orgasm—was the source of health and renewal for human beings. Resistence to orgasmic release perverted humanity, creating isolation, indigence, a craving for authority, and mystic longing (Reich 1978: 4). Reich was the harbinger of sexual freedom and "natural morality" (1978: 14). The free expression of the sexual bioenergy was his primary goal. For modern Neo-Reichians, in-terpersonal and small group breathing exercises and body work are the keys to this release (Kelley and Wright n.d.).

Reich's ethos was curiously echoed by Hugh Hefner, cited by sev-eral informants as a source of inspiration. Initially, this association was perplexing, but *Playboy*'s rampant sensuality and individual ex-pression were consistent with the search for sexual energy. Hefner pro-moted an attractive life-style that joined values and behavior, along with freedom from convention. Bhagwan Shree Rajneesh, the eclectic Indian teacher, whose devoted sunyasi followers have made their way into holistic health circles, also promoted the orgasmic vision. Practic-ing an ecstatic dancing meditation and promoting the free expression of sexuality, his orange and purple clad disciples raise their energy lev-els to cosmic heights. Ironically enough, this would have undoubtedly offended Reich, who saw all mystic longing as a suppression of the sexual energy (1973: 92–93; 1978: 322).

Reich was correct in perceiving that there was a long tradition in turning the rising sexual ecstacy into a mystical conduit. The practice of suppressing the climax of sexual behavior and transforming that urge to spirituality was used by tantric believers, early Christian Gnos-tics (Walker 1983: 114–20), and by the modern theurgist, Aleister Crowley in his "sex magick." The aim was to increase sexual energy, but suppress physical release, driving the energy inward and upward. The "new celibacy" of the polarity practitioners is a classic expression of this practice. The newly released orgone/ kundalini energy is re-channeled into spiritual concerns. This practice promotes sexual awareness and ecstacy, often through pain and emotional catharsis, but for a very non-Reichian goal.

The ecstatic states of the Reichians, polarity therapists, and the meditative revery of individual holistic health practitioners reflect a tra-dition of shamanistic trance. The cognitive content of that trance can be learned in the small group, with acknowledgement and praise rein-forcing the special perception. It would be foolish to overlook the ob-vious, that the body itself may provide its own reinforcement for al-tered states of consciousness. Unfortunately, most of the research on altered states of consciousness has been purely ethnographic, not psy-chobiological (Bourguigon 1973: 13). The precise psychophysical na-ture of that trance remains unknown, but there are several interesting lines of study.

The altered state of a shaman, and by extension a holistic healer, could be traced through one of two known psychological and somatic mechanisms: hypnosis and ubiquitous endorphins (Prince 1982). Hypnosis appears to be a separate phenomenon from endorphin produced states. Hypnosis is not usually prevented by the endorphin antagonist, naloxone (Pomeranz 1982: 387; Prince 1982: 411), although this has been known (Jilek 1982: 340). Hypnosis also has an ambiguous relationship to the placebo effect, sometimes reinforcing the effect but occasionally showing no contritution to the role of the placebo. (Orne 1980: 154–92; Prince 1982: 471). Hypnosis is related to some kinds of meditation, such as biofeedback techniques using autogenic training (Pelletier 1977: 229–33) but not zazen, Zen Buddhist sitting/breathing meditation. (1977: 199). Contradictory experimental evidence and the lack of field studies make it difficult to assess the contribution of hypnosis to the altered state of shamans. Within the holistic health community, hypnosis and self-hypnosis are seen as powerful tools and are sought as paths of insight and control. Mail order tapes, workshops, and literature abound.

Speculation has run rampant about the possibility that endorphins may be the mechanism for an altered state of consciousness. Endorphins regulate pain and temperature, influence perceptions of pleasure and mood, regulate drives (Cotman and McGaugh 1980: 243), and if produced after an event, enhance the long-term memory of that event (Stein and Bellozzi 1979: 383–85). They produce tremors, similar to the phenomenon of trance trembling (Henry 1982: 404). Endorphins, like hypnosis, have been linked to the placebo effect (Levine, Gordon and Fields 1978).

Endorphins can be induced through a variety of actions, all having implications for holistic health clients and practitioners. The most obvious link to alternative healing is through acupuncture induced analgesia. Acupuncture stimulation is hypothesized to produce endorphins, which then block the sensation of pain (G. Chen 1975; G. S. Chen 1977; Chung and Dickenson 1980; Henry 1982: 404; Peng, Yang, Kok and Woo 1978; Pomeranz 1982; Tappan 1978; Yang and Kok 1979). The hypothesis has been tested along various lines of evidence. Experiments either transfer blood serum from untreated and treated animals and test for resistence to pain (Tappan 1978) or explore the differences between known and bogus acupuncture points (Pomeranz 1982). It has been noted that: 1) Endorphin blocking drugs (naloxone) block acupuncture effectiveness; 2) Reduction of pituitary hormones decreases acupuncture effectiveness; 3) Endorphins are released into cerebrospinal fluid during electro-acupuncture treatments; and 4) Genetic lack of an endorphin system prevents the acupuncture effect from occurring (Pomeranz 1982: 391).

The effects of acupuncture build up slowly from thirty to sixty minutes and continue for thirty to sixty minutes (Pomeranz 1982: 389; Yang and Kok 1979). It is difficult to assess whether all alternative explanations have been eliminated, yet the possibility of endorphin release in acupuncture clearly has implications for holistic health practitioners. Manipulation of acupuncture points is common to most body work. As trainee clients, practitioners may learn to sense the endorphin-induced altered state of consciousness. Other mechanisms of endorphin production may be invoked by the practitioner to regain this state.

Stress (Henry 1982: 404; Prince 1982: 412), excitation of proprioceptive receptors—that is, internally generated physical conditions—vigorous motor activity, pain, emotive hyperstress (Prince 1982 414), extended sensory input (1982: 414), and suggestion (Henry 1982: 405) all play a part in producing endorphins. Any of these conditions could conceivably be used to induce an alternative consciousness in the body of the practitioner during a therapeutic session.

Field evidence is utterly absent, but the possibility of an endorphin/hypnosis mechanism for practitioner/shamanistic trance suggests several potential lines of research. Does the client, in a therapeutic session, show clinical signs of hypnosis (as shown on a electroencephalograph) or increased endorphin levels? The tremors, euphoria, and drive changes in the more dramatic therapies would suggest that this is a strong possibility. Does either hypnosis or endorphin production really apply to the practitioner? Above all, does the act of experiencing an altered state of consciousness as a client enable the practitioner to learn to change his/her own consciousness by inducing self-hypnosis or the production of endorphins?

EMBODYING THE MOVEMENT

In this chapter, I have been concerned with the minute internal states of the individual practitioner within the movement. For the purposes of understanding a social movement, it is more fruitful to look at the psychology of learning, not abnormality. From the moment a person decides to enter the movement as a practitioner, not just a client, he/she has decisions to make and information to learn. That initial choice may be based on ideology or a personal experience as a client. Rarely, after the fashion of the shaman, it may even be perceived as an involuntary calling. Learning to become a practitioner is an extension of the role of the client.

Inspired by books, intuition, and teachers, the novice learns techniques, the Aquarian moral code, and a new style of thinking. The novice develops an internal world view, tested and reinforced by self-knowledge and interaction within the small group. Interaction with the client is particularly valuable as a learning tool, though the kinds of rapport may vary widely. Ultimately, the novice must learn to develop a special cognitive style, a highly controlled altered perception. An empirical healer uses the vital force and the ability to perceive and control this force as the source of the healing medium—energy and the route to personal growth and safety.

The special perception of the holistic health practitioner bears a resemblance to the milder forms of shamanistic trance. Like shamanism, the trances can vary from meditation to ecstatic revelations. Empathy and close rapport promote a meditative state, while invoked sexuality produces a more dramatic reaction in the client. These states are experienced intensively as a client-in-training and then with more control as a practitioner. I have only seen these states expressed in the most obvious form, noticable to an ethnographer. The subtleties of experiment, particularly neurophysiological experiment, are absent. However, recent studies linking altered states of consciousness with hypnosis and endorphins suggests some interesting research possibilities.

From the level of individual neurochemistry to the responses of peer, client, and teacher, the novice practitioner embodies the values of the social movement. To be effective as a social movement, individual behavior must be integrated with the society. For the holistic health practitioner, effectiveness means creating a professional niche. As the groups learn to be politically and legally competent, they begin to professionalize. This process includes establishing generalized areas of knowledge, forming standards of ethics that are self-policed, and developing a sense of obligation towards the community (Jackson 1970: 8). In holistic health, this means standardizing training, licensing practitioners, and establishing a separate legal identity. This is the focus of chapter 7.

SHAMAN OR PROFESSIONAL?

Redundancy . . . is our main
avenue of survival. (*Shadrach in*
the Furnace, Silverberg 1976: 4)

Personal choices shape varied, complex societies, and the individual options are in turn molded by social forces. Novice healers are exposed to an overall binding value system, but within that system they are free to create unique personal styles of empirical practice. Once the decision to go from client to practitioner is made, he/she is launched on a dynamic course of yet more decisions. Should legal restrictions be changed or ignored? Is there an advantage to becoming "professional?" Will this shift in social status improve the position of the holistic health movement or will it compromise the basic values? What does professionalization imply? To what extent should orthodox medicine be recognized? All these questions play a part in the choices envisioned by the holistic health practitioner.

The choices conceived by the holistic health community were revealed in daily discussion, life histories, and especially the projection of ethnographic futures. Bright visions of medical plurality contrast with fears of complete absorption into the medical establishment or alternatively, a return to underground status. Practitioners' futures will be examined in terms of the available choices. Each choice is linked to other factors in the society. Complementing social movements promote the survival of holistic health as a viable entity, just as others fosters visions of control and authority.

For example, women, often the most powerless health care consumers, were particularly supportive of holistic health. Familial and life crises, births, and deaths were of minimal concern in orthodox medicine, but were central in holistic health. Even in the history of holistic health, there is a connection between the woman's political control of her body and empirical medicine. As a self-medication, the nostrum, Lydia Pinkham's Vegetable Compound, was a "blow for women's rights" during the 1870s, freeing them from insensitive male physicians" (Young 1977: 100). In Paraiso and the Bay Area, feminist psychotherapy and female-only practices echo this sentiment (Mattson 1982: 67). Certainly much in the movement toward natural childbirth in America has paralleled the attitudes of holistic health. Midwives I have interviewed stressed such holistic values as the introduction of an element of spirituality, a more mother-centered practice, and greater client responsibility. These ideas persist in spite of enormous pressure to medicalize, that is, to conform to hospital birthing practices, to reduce the amount of client-midwife interaction, and to increase medical intervention.

Immediate survival goals might limit options, creating a social trap. The inherent individualism of the movement, and the need for an identity distinct from orthodox medicine, make it difficult to organize and enter the world of professionals. There are still ways out of such a social trap. I will consider the possibilities available to practitioners as a social group. Finally, I will consider the position that social movements are the media for making the decisions of the past become the plans of the future, wherein the wishes and decisions of an individual shape his society.

NEW CAREER OR SPURIOUS PROFESSIONAL?

The nature of the relationship between client and practitioner opens the holistic health community to charges of spurious and marginal professionalism. If a practitioner is guided more by client feedback than his peers, he falls under the sociological definition of quackery (Cobb 1977: 10–11). This is not, however, as straightforward as it would first seem. The holistic health movement has not been developing in a vacuum. Other social movements have flourished since the 1960s, promoting so called new careers that are based on humanistic values. Two separate social forces either condone or condemn the empathic/ empirical therapeutic relationship.

In the 1960s and early 1970s, a profusion of social movements emerged, focused on consciousness raising and personal behavior, consumer rights, ecology, community action and women's and civil rights. Spurred on by catalytic analysts—Ralph Nader, Martin Luther King and so forth—the movements were promoted by widespread media attention and helped shape American values (Platt 1975). They advocated individual rights, creativity, and decentralization. These movements could never hope to take on established institutions except by individual change and informal networks. At the same time, for every move toward individual freedom, there were countermovements focusing on greater efficiency, centralization, and authority. America has experienced "law-and-order" movements as well as human rights and human potential. As the research of Marchetti (1985) points out, recent movements, such as the charismatic movement, are actively seeking authority, producing organizations and centralization. Both sets of values, individualistic and authoritarian, have an impact on the holistic health movement.

The devaluation of patient/client assessment of health care as quackery, only makes sense if the client is perceived as ignorant and passive. In the past, this described the image of the American consumer. The 1960s revolt of the consumer was devoted to changing this perception. In the health care industry, consumer rights rapidly evolved into patient's rights. The idea of the patient as a responsible human being led individuals into a natural alliance with holistic health (Mattson 1982: 67; Roth 1976: 34, 122–23).

Pristine nature, a diminishing commodity in modern America, became a matter of attention and value as a result of the ecological movement. Natural cures and natural food fit into this value system nicely (see Mattson 1982: 65; Roth 1976: 122–23). These values directly contributed to the renaissance of chiropractic in the 1960s (Cobb 1977: 14), health food (Mattson 1982: 65), and the wealth of "organic" materia medica available to holistic practitioners. The focus on the sanctity of nature came with the human potential movement, promoting self-actualization and fullfillment.

The combination of consumerism, ecological awareness, and human liberation movements produced new careers that valued socio-emotive skills such as empathy, personal involvement, and experiential knowledge (Cobb 1977: 15) over purely technical skills. Holistic health could fit under the rubric of new careers creating a niche that does not have to conform to classical definitions of professionalism. The values that permit the creation of new careers, are probably not the guidelines for those who control the legislatures, the insurance companies, or the universities that lend legitimacy to any aspiring health care niche. The conflicts typified by the second century orthodox church and the Gnostics, or the empirical practitioners of the 1850s and the newborn A.M.A., are again played out in the struggle between authoritative structure and individual expression. Holistic health, despite individual allies within the orthodox medical world, is not part of the elite. In fact, for its own initial survival, it needed to compete with that elite.

As a complex system expands, it develops maintenance goals beyond the initial purpose. The growth of holistic health as a social entity led to behavior that promotes identity formation and survival. That growth runs counter to the survival goals of orthodox medicine. Each system of healing, empirical and rationalist, has developed a set of rules designed primarily to promote its own survival. Each needed to define itself more clearly to exclude the other—one was science, the other humanism.

Holistic health seeks to reinstate traditional healing techniques and the underpinning belief in a reality that extends beyond the material. Holistic health fosters the art and craft of healing, taught best by close individual interaction and by experience. This promotes a sense of tradition. On the other hand, orthodox medicine is based on informational growth and the pursuit of cause in a materialistic paradigm. Being "objective," it can be learned from an outside source and is not utterly dependent on experience. In a practice, the holistic healer must make it clear to the client that he/she is not practicing rationalist medicine or any part of it. Otherwise, she is practicing medicine without a license. The severity of the consequences accelerates the creation of the distinction. Bateson called this process schismogenesis—the generation of behavioral differences through individual interaction (1958: 175, 285–90). This interaction is guided by locked-in patterns. For instance, driving on the right side of the road, precludes driving on the left, minimizing chaos (Platt 1969; 1980). Once a pattern is set, it limits the choices available.

To protect its turf, medicine must define itself to include as much as possible. To escape this definition, any alternative system must define itself as narrowly as possible outside orthodox medicine. In the beginning, this is a wise strategy—orthodox medicine was unmoved by the intrusion of an upstart fad. Holistic health was distinct enough to infringe only minimally on the practice of medicine. This advantage is ultimately illusory, however. It was a sliding reinforcement. What was good in the beginning precluded the long-term payoff and became a social trap (Platt 1973: 664). At the same time, to establish a separate identity, holistic health has had to define itself vis-à-vis orthodox medicine. This is another aspect of the social trap. By taking on the medical Goliath, holistic health risks the danger of being dismissed by them as spurious. The marginal category means being conversant in professional trappings, but not really meeting the criteria of professionalism as defined by sociologists, lawyers, and the American Medical Association.

If holistic health is at odds with the establishment, it cannot professionalize. Natural hygiene, conceptually and verbally at odds with the world of the M.D., is a choice illustration. By perceiving drugs as poison, and physicians as insidious promoters of ill health, natural hygienists make their conflict clear (Diamond 1979; Roth 1976: 15, 58). Speaking of the history of orthodox medicine, one hygienist flatly stated, "You'd think it was all an incredible plot." No matter what the appeal of the therapy of natural hygiene, the polemics in Paraiso eventually alienated the "soldiers." Novices began to avoid the zealous practitioner/teacher. Novices were uncomfortable faced with this bias. How can the movement grow if it takes on the Goliath medical establishment? The novices discussed how difficult it would be to present those ideas to clients and certainly to valuable professional allies.

On the other hand, if holistic health practitioners try to make overtures at peace and cooperation, they run the risk of being absorbed. Osteopathy, in the United States, has become increasingly acceptable to the American medical world by becoming part of it. Efforts to regain distinction must now fight those osteopaths who have become part of the orthodoxy. Homeopathy almost met the same fate, but the promoters of Hahnemann's high potency (spiritual) remedies fought the co-option, even though it meant loss of institutional support (Kaufman 1971: 175–85). By creating a solution to the short-term legal problem, holistic health has created a long-term professional quandary. Neither competition nor cooperation can yield the desired scheme of medical plurality.

The "holistic physician" is a prime illustration of this conflict. Trained and allied with the rationalist paradigm, he attempts to incorporate empiricist techniques. As a result, he is a heretic, an offshoot of the medical world. He may be actively distrusted by some novices and practitioners. Holistic health practitioners believe themselves to be perceived by holistic physicians as ancillary specialists at best, if not a legacy to be left behind. The internal friction generated by the social trap locks holistic health practitioners into few alternatives.

The second inherent social trap is the promotion of individuality and personal experience. Some practitioners do not want to organize. The freedom that they experience, especially as lay practitioners, is what drew them to the movement. Joining organizations and becoming established is not what they sought. It was what they were leaving. The individualism of the early Gnostics and the Theosophists created perpetual fission, thriving in informal networks of allies until a new vision came along. Similarly, Doug—a pioneer in Paraiso's holistic health community—having rebelled against his establishment life, was resistant to professionalization. He wanted no "organic fascists" to interfere with his practice or his life-style. With a motto of "eat cookies and drink beer," he exemplified the individualism basic to the young holistic health movement. Even ideology would not lock him into a pattern. Those that promote professionalism recognize that networks, organizations, and standards will be necessary—but at the cost of individual free expression.

In professional holistic health, creativity and experiential learning are still encouraged, but within a framework of organization. Patrick, a leader of professional holistic health practitioners in Paraiso, works ceaselessly for the creation of a holistic health community and the transformation of that community into a profession. He promotes syntheses, urging practitioners to learn rationalist science and to create professional and credible "health enhancement." In light of the social traps, how would this synthesis occur? If the practitioners cannot safely compete or cooperate with orthodox medicine, how can they institutionalize? Is institutionalization the same as survival?

ANTICIPATED HEALTH CARE
SCENARIOS

My observation of holistic health practitioners and use of the EFR technique revealed a concern for integration with the entire society. By anticipating future medical practice, holistic healers discuss the topics that will influence their economic and social vitality in the next twenty-five years. Two dominant themes emerged. Practitioners would prefer to practice in the empirical tradition, as professionals in their own right, working in an atmosphere of medical plurality. At the same time, they fear this will not be so. Perhaps they will be swallowed by the powerful medical establishment, so that only synthetic holistic M.D.s could practice. These M.D.s would be neither wholly rationalist nor empirical. The empirical practitioners would have no choice but to be laymen, going underground.

Involvement with orthodox medicine and governmental licensing loom large in the EFR scenarios and in holistic health community discussions. Favored futures focus on a free health care market, with medical plurality as the rule. The degree to which future professionalism in holistic health is based on the "medical model" is a source of variation in EFR interviews and a point of contention in the community. Concerning practice, best case scenarios focus on developing a cooperative but autonomous relationship with orthodox medicine. In the optimistic scenario, holistic healers do not exclude cosmopolitan medicine. They hope the need for any disease care itself will be minimal. The practitioner's attitude toward medical science is parallel to Gandhi's desire for a synthesis of Ayurvedic, Unani, and cosmopolitan medicine. He admired the spirit of science, but not its directions, and hoped to combine the rigor and availability of science with the ethics and ecological focus of Indian medicine (Gandhi 1978: 8–9). Technology is to be used "appropriately" and allopathic medicine limited to physical trauma and acute conditions.

The thrust of research will be on empirical examination since no causative agent can be isolated and researcher rapport is a vital factor. Vital to this scenario is autonomy for holistic health practitioners. They must be separate and equal to medical physicians (Green 1978b: 4–6). They also hope for social and legal institutions that clearly support holistic health.

Worst case scenarios invariably include conquest by the medical community, leaving holistic health practitioners without a real or legal identity. There is a fear of being swallowed, losing important components of holistic health to "medical" practitioners. Practitioners believe that orthodox medicine distrusts the psychic and spiritual aspects of holistic health and its philosophical biases against the reality of "objective science" (Mattson 1982: 158–59). Holistic health practitioners foresee a dual fate. Those who resist absorption into cosmopolitan medicine, or practice in fields too alien from it will be forced underground, and will fade from public view. Others will become "holistic medical practitioners," adopting the bedside manner of the holistic healer, but not the core of assumptions and goals that make it viable as a distinct option. These "heretics" will be most avid in suppressing the remnants of alternative medicine.

"Staying on purpose" to maintain professional identity and integrity is the primary variable for the future of holistic health practice. There are practical constraints that influence the most probable scenario. Licensing is ambiguous. To practice openly in the community a holistic healer must either be a suspect "massage parlour prostitute," act as a religious practitioner, or walk the thin edge of practicing "medicine" without a license.

Faced with such ideas, imitating the professional trappings of orthodox health practices can be seen as one practical solution for staying out of trouble. However, it is also seen as the road to the dissolution of the movement, losing those cross-cultural and "spiritual" elements that distinguish holistic health from orthodox medicine.

These issues are brought to bear in daily life through choices of licensing, advertising, and public education. Such individual choices are perceived as crucial to the future of holistic health practice. There is a conscious political effort to accord "holistic health practitioner" and related professions legal status of their own, not just accepting marginal roles of masseur, nurse, religious counselor or being tied to a physician for legitimation. Consumer education through classes, workshops, and advertising are critical in developing this identity. This means not only instructing people about acupuncture, homeopathy, diet, and so forth but teaching the larger Aquarian promise. The difference "between a liberal doctor" and a holistic health practitioner is commitment to spiritual transformation (Grossinger 1980: 339) and the empirical approach.

In chapter 2, I made the distinction between the sub-rosa, lay practitioner and the emerging professional holistic health practitioner in Paraiso. In the link between individual and society—the choice of whether to be professional—is a critical one. Even though the lay healer and the holistic health professional may have read the same books, gone through the same workshops, and even practiced identical techniques, there is an immense social difference. The distinctions in social organization, limitations, and potentials influence the shape of the entire holistic health movement.

A lay healer is not necessarily poorly qualified or illegal, but is a practitioner who, by choice, practices within a small preestablished network—friends, fellow church goers, engineers, nurses, or kin. He or she may even be licensed, although there is no ready way to know the percentage that make that choice. They may be highly skilled, or not—ultimately that decision is in the hands of the client. Even if highly qualified, they may reject institutional constraints of licensure and formal organizations. Much as some have rejected organized religion, the laymen reject organized professionalism. Disgust at the negative sanctions wrought by degrading massage and "quack" laws and the desire to stay outside "the system" influence this decision. Whatever the initial reason, the practitioners stay in contact only through egalitarian peer groups and continuing educational workshops.

In the informal setting, the lay practitioners provide a powerful informal educational base for the movement. Lay practitioners were the basis of empirical medicine for centuries before the renaissance of Paracelsus. It is difficult to eliminate a diffuse and invisible network. At the same time, power is limited. The ability to lobby for more reputable laws, gain open social recognition for the movement, or even make a profitable living are impaired. Moreover, lay practitioners cannot be regulated. This may be a motivation for the individualistic layman, but it also means that there is no quality control. Naturally, this reflects on the movement. Kevin and Barbara Kunz, professional reflexologists reflect that "for every oddity out there practicing reflexology, it takes ten serious professionals to offset the damage done to the image" (1982: 74).

A social movement can provide the basis for the creation of a professional identity. There are two aspects to professionalism, community and formal organization (Turner and Hodge 1970: 32). A social movement is designed to build a community with shared values and skills. It may develop into an institution. Witness the formation of the Catholic Church, discussed in chapter 5. For the holistic health movement, professionalism is the direction sought for institutionalization.

Activities new to the social movement are necessary in creating a profession. The cycle of professionalization begins with full-time activity, followed by the establishment of schools (Pavalko 1971: 29).

Holistic health is just now creating accredited academies. In an attempt to change images, newborn professions may decide to change the name of their occupation, projecting an image of increased competence and prestige (Pavalko 1971: 28). In holistic health, the word *healer* conjures an image of faith and charisma. Practitioner or therapist are preferred titles. This process is ideally followed by the creation of professional associations, political agitation to create a legal niche, and the development of ethical codes (Pavalko 1971: 29). Ethics are a strong point in holistic health; it is a movement born of humanistic concerns. However, lobbying is difficult without a financial base, although legal expertise is not lacking within the holistic health movement (Green 1974; 1978).

The limitation in creating a profession stems from the diverse nature and ethos of individualism in holistic health. Established organizations, such as the American Massage Therapy Association, serve as an umbrella organization for body work practitioners, but they are of little help to herbalists. The American Holistic Medical Association represents the interests of holistic physicians only. The National Health Federation, frequently promotional, rather than professional, lacks the base to become the encompassing organization. New organizations were created to contain the diversity of holistic health. The creation of a Holistic Health Practitioners Association was not successful because internal divisions were too great. It was followed by the California Health Practitioners Association, but no widespread organizational commitment existed among practitioners.

The lack of formal organization makes it difficult to implement the characteristics of a developed profession. A synthesized list of these characteristics includes: 1) Lifelong commitment; 2) Mastery of a body of knowledge; 3) Formal and lengthy training; 4) Control of licensing; 5) Control of educational requirements; 6) Internal policing; 7) Control of legal scope of work; and 8) Possession of mechanisms for legal, economic, and political survival. (Lewis and Maude 1952: 55–66; Maykovich 1980; 267–71; and Unschuld 1979: 5). The greater the degree of compliance to this list, the higher the social status. This definition is epitomized by the cosmopolitan medical profession, which was the model for the list. Without a formal encompassing organization, these components are difficult to master. Lacking this power base, holistic health practitioners attempt to create a professional image at the individual level. This is done in four ways: creating a sense of business acumen, professional environment, ethical guidelines, and increased standards of competence and responsibility.

The ability to create and maintain a business is the border between lay and professional practice. Retail sales of exercise equipment, vitamins, herbs, and various new age paraphernalia are links to potential clients. Education is the key to gaining and keeping clients. Creative business cards, brochures, and journal articles are avenues for gaining clients. Novices are told to become speakers or workshop teachers, join voluntary organizations, and create networks. Practitioners are directed to get involved with the community, especially the well educated, for they make the best clients and converts.

Kunz and Kunz, in advising professional reflexologists, suggest that the business establishment should be clean and orderly and should present an air of authority and stability (1982: 74, 86). For the holistic health practitioner in Paraiso, this is not always the case. The local massage laws have many restrictions on the location of a professional office. For example, it cannot be near a school, for the establishment is seen as the legal equivalent of a "massage parlor," a source of corruption to young and vulnerable minds. In addition, the enormous overhead of renting any real estate in this coastal paradise is prohibitive. Most practitioners are lucky to able to find a place to live, let alone rent a business site. As a consequence, practitioners feel it wisest to get a license that allows practice in the client's home. This means that the practitioner herself must project an image of cleanliness, stability, and competence.

The novices are told to dress conservatively, perhaps using organic fibers, but not obviously counterculturally. Cleanliness, promptness, and respectfulness are virtues to be cultivated by the practitioner. In practice, simple techniques such as making and keeping appointments are encouraged. Letting the client "drop in" or make unreasonable time demands is said to lead to diminished professionalism. Respect is to be earned by keeping a relationship professional and projecting self-confidence through increased prices and professional demeanor.

Ethics are particularly important in a field where images of sleazy massage parlors and snake oil salesmen are retained in the popular imagination. Within the holistic health community, there is a strong feeling of puritanism. Sexual conduct is separate from business. If seduction occurs, then it is not business and money should never be exchanged. Only two informants protested this attitude, both male. Advertisements reflect this attitude. "Nonsexual" and "ethical" massage are the linguistic markers between professional body workers and the pleasure palace and massage parlor.

Responsibility toward the client is paramount. Dishonesty and promises of a panacea are not allowed. Effort is spent to drill this idea into the minds of the novices. Holistic health balances energy and promotes healthful living of "clients," it does not cure "patients." The novices are warned against promising cures or even using the words diagnosis and cure. The "science of pathology" is medicine—orthodox, legally powerful, medicine. Only honesty about the principles and limitations of empirical techniques are safeguards against "practicing medicine without a license." The practitioners must act responsibly toward clients, telling them about the unpleasant possibility of a healing crises, keeping records, making contracts, and insuring that the clients' expectations are practical (Kunz and Kunz 1982: 75–86). Ultimately, an unhappy client is the source of legal headaches. A happy client is the source of potential professional status—a goal in the holistic health movement.

THE SURVIVAL OF HOLISTIC HEALTH

For holistic health, redundancy may be the avenue of survival. Several variables may change which will permit holistic health to survive as a professional entity. By changing the thrust of the movement, becoming reformative, not revolutionary, holistic health may exist as a form of specialized holistic medicine. Holistic health may be able to create its own legal and professional niche, working with orthodox medicine, as psychologists and clergy now work with the medical establishment. These categories, however, will not contain those who are firmly immersed in the individuality and identity of alternative healers. Those individuals can practice in the already existant category of informal lay practitioners. They represent a noninstitutionalized avenue of survival, typical of the empirical healing and mystical traditions for many centuries. Whether as holistic medical practitioners, holistic health practitioners, or lay healers, the movement can only continue to function in an atmosphere of medical plurality.

Medical plurality refers to the existence of several separate medical traditions within the same society. Most of the anthropological studies of medical plurality have been outside the developed countries—in China (Crozier 1976; Unschuld 1976), India (Leslie 1975; 1976b), and of course, a variety of examinations concerning indigenous healers in Latin America, Africa, and the Pacific. In this context, indigenous healing represents a form of national pride for the Third World. Traditional medical systems exist side by side with attempts to introduce large-scale orthodox health programs. These are different phenomena from medical plurality in the developed countries, where the movements are revivals of imported or historic systems of healing existing in an arena already clearly dominated by orthodox medicine.

Otsuka's study of the revival of kanpo, Chinese medicine in Japan (1976), Cobb's investigation of chiropractic in the United States (1977), and Roth's study of the natural health movement in both the United States and Germany (1976) indicate that there is another process that leads to medical plurality in the developed world. In Japan, Germany, and the United States, disatisfaction with the rationalist, materialist model and the perceived lack of interpersonal empathy by orthodox medicine has provided fuel for medical revivals. The nationalistic medical revivals in the Third World have increased the exposure of the developed countries to naturalistic medical systems, especially from China and India (Otsuka 1976: 338–39). Even though historic empirical tradition existed in those countries, their resurgence took place after the rationalist medical system was firmly rooted. The direction of the survival of holistic health depends on the legal niche left by the orthodox medical world.

Orthodox medicine will not necessarily steadfastly stick to its own current identity—especially if consumers (that is, patients) demand a greater emphasis on holistic health. As this occurs, the legal niche of orthodox medicine might increase to crowd out the competitors. If the definition of the practice of medicine is widened to include "health enhancement" as well as the science of pathology, then holistic health will have to become holistic medicine. It will be reborn as a medical reform rather than a transformative vision. Even if the definition is not broadened, practitioners are anticipating this change and are now entering or returning to the orthodox medical occupations, with the intent to reform. The basic principles of holism and compassion will remain, along with some of the imported techniques of acupuncture and manipulation (Snyder 1980: 2–4), but the Neoplatonic themes of microcosm and energetic body will probably be submerged. The "holistic physician," rightly perceived as threat to the Aquarian egalitarian vision, will become the norm for this avenue of professional survival.

The professional alternative to this is the creation of a niche for practitioners of empirical medicine. This can only happen if the orthodox medical world does not define its scope of work to include health enhancement. To some extent, this niche already exists for chiropractors, and in fewer states, for acupunturists and naturopaths. Such professions must struggle to keep their own niches, and cannot extend them to embrace other practitioners of holistic health without threatening their own legal stability. The creation of the holistic health practitioner niche in Paraiso is an example of what can be done. They neither diagnose pathology nor treat it. They do not practice rationalist medicine (Green 1974: 19–20; Kunz and Kunz 1982: 75). They may embrace psychic, physical, and emotional therapies that promote self-understanding and self-healing by the client. In other words, they still define their identity vis-à-vis orthodox medicine. There is, however, a subtle change.

The promoters of the new professionalism, also emphasize complementing, not competing with, orthodox medicine. They resist absorption but also direct conflict (Kunz and Kunz 1982: 86). The closer the therapy is to "religious" and metaphysical concepts, the easier it is to avoid competition from the perspective of the practitioner. Skultans' study of Spiritualists in South Wales suggests that the practitioners see their role as complementary to the medical establishment (1976: 196–97). Alice Bailey, a catalyst for psychic healing, also recommends cooperation with the materialist physicians. In her view, practitioners would become specialists in integrating spiritual concerns (Bailey 1980: 254).

To justify the new professional image, some internal policing would be necessary. Just as the National Health Federation has needed to limit some of the more "outlandish" claims to increase its legitimacy (Roth 1976: 27–33, 68), some weeding would have to take place. Professionalizing holistic health practitioners recognize this, just as individualists like the charismatic Doug reject it. Some of the goals of a movement may not be amenable to bureaucratization (Ash and Zald 1969: 484).

Holistic health may function as a professionally separate entity, or it may exist as reformed orthodoxy. Once again, however, legitimation must not be confused with survival. Even though the early Christian Valentinian Gnostics were unsuccessful at synthesis or establishing their own church, they survived as individuals in informal, decentralized nodes. Their ideas were repeatedly adopted by mystics and heretics for centuries. The plethora of lay practitioners, trained but not public, create a source of continued existence, in spite of any action of the establishment. Legally protected by "freedom of religion," or simply hidden from the eyes of the establishment, lay practitioners can keep learning, teaching, fissioning, and practicing within small informal networks. Such survival is the crowning benefit of belonging to an informal network. It cannot easily be controlled or destroyed (Ferguson 1980: 217; Gerlach and Hine 1981: 66–77; Hine 1977: 19). Lay practitioners cannot organize, advertise, or get insurance or tax breaks, but they can still practice their craft outside the system.

The holistic health movement, dedicated to individuality and empirical medicine, had to create a unique sociological niche. This niche, though necessary, also created impediments to professionalization. Utterly dependent on a position defined by the dominant medical establishment, the holistic health practitioners had the choice of becoming absorbed as medical reformers or placed in a narrowly defined role. However, professionalism and the creation of institutions are not the only definitions of survival: the practitioners may continue the tradition of lay practice, maintaining the goals and traditions of empirical medicine. It is a matter of individual choice.

This work represents only the tip of the iceberg. The complex relationships in professional and client networks, the myriad array of beliefs and practices, are far more intricate than I could possibly convey. There are many more intriguing issues to explore. My major concern was with practitioners, but who are the clients? Why do they use holistic health and when? How well does it work for them? My information was regional, based on the practitioners of Southern California. Paraiso had legal niches for chiropractors, acupuncturists, and holistic health practitioners but not for naturopaths. How do holistic health practices vary within the United States? How does the local variation in law and licensing influence the nature of the holistic health community? Although some studies have been conducted in Japan and Germany, how does traditional medicine fare in other developed countries? The act of balancing traditional and Western orthodox medicine is a daily occurrence in places like China, where traditional medicine gets official support, or Mexico, where it does not. How does legality and public respect influence the continuity of Asian or Mexican Hippocratic medical traditions? Do syntheses with modern medicine come easier in China because the need to resist cooptation is low? These questions are not only for social scientists to consider but also for practitioners, who need to see that their practices are part of a much greater dynamic of medical plurality on a varied and intricate planet.

R E F E R E N C E S
C   I   T   E   D

Aberle, David
    1962   A Note on the Relative Deprivation Theory as Applied to Millenarian
    and other Cult Movements. *In* Millenial Dreams in Action: Essays in
    Comparative Study. Comparative Studies in Society and History, Suppl. 2.
    Sylvia Thrupp, ed. Pp. 209–14. The Hague: Mouton and Company.
Academy of Traditional Chinese Medicine
    1975   An Outline of Chinese Acupuncture. Peking: Foreign Language
    Press.
Addison, C. G.
    1978   The Knights Templar History. New York: AMS Press.
Agar, Michael
    1980   The Professional Stranger. New York: Academic Press.
Agren, Hans
    1975   A New Approach to Chinese Traditional Medicine. American Journal
    of Chinese Medicine. 3(3): 207–12.
Ahlstrom, Sydney
    1978   From Sinai to the Golden Gate: The Liberation of Religion in the Oc-
    cident. *In* Understanding the New Religions. Jacob Needleman and
    George Bakers, eds. Pp. 3–22. New York: Seabury Press.
Albus, James
    1981   Brains, Behavior and Robotics. Peterborough, N.H.: Byte Books,
    Subsidiary of McGraw-Hill.
Albon, Joan
    1977   Field Method in Working with Middle Class Americans: New Issues of
    Values, Personality and Reciprocity. Human Organization 36(1): 69–72.
Albanese, Catherine L.
    1977   Corresponding Motion: Transcendental Religion and the New Amer-
    ica. Philadelphia: Temple University Press.
Alexander, Thea
    1976   2150 A.D. Tempe, Arizona: Macro Books.
American Herbal Pharmacology Delegation
    1975   Herbal Pharmacology in the People's Republic of China. Washing-
    ton: National Academy of Sciences.
Anderson, David
    1979   Homeopathic Remedies for Physicians, Laymen and Therapists.
    Homesdale, PA: Himalayan International Institute of Yoga, Science and
    Philosophy.

Ash, Roberta and Mayer Zald
    1969   Social Movement Organizations: Growth, Decay and Change. *In*
        Studies in Social Movements: A Social Psychological Perspective. Barry
        McLaughlin, ed. Pp. 461–85. New York: The Free Press.
Asthana, Shashi
    1976   History and Archaeology of India's Contacts with Other Countries,
        from Earliest Times to 300 B.C. Delhi: B. R. Publishing Corporation.
Bach, Richard
    1984   Illusions: the Adventures of a Reluctant Messiah. New York: Dell
        Publishing.
Bailey, Alice
    1980   Esoteric Healing. New York: Lucis Publishing Company.
Baker, Elsworth, and Arthur Nelson
    1981   Orgone Therapy. *In* Handbook of Innovative Psychotherapies.
        Raymond Corsini, ed. Pp. 599–612. New York: Wiley-Interscience Pub-
        lications.
Ballentine, Rudolph
    1979   Diet and Nutrition: A Holistic Approach. Homesdale, PA: The Hima-
        layan International Institute.
Barkun, Michael
    1974   Disaster and the Millenium. New Haven, CT: Yale University Press.
Barnstone, Willis
    1984   The Other Bible. San Francisco: Harper and Row.
Barraclough, Geoffrey
    1982   The Times Concise Atlas of World History. Maplewood, NJ: Ham-
        mond Incorporated.
Basham, A. L.
    1977   The Practice of Medicine in Ancient and Medieval India. *In* Asian
        Medical Systems. Charles Leslie, ed. Pp. 18–43. Berkeley: University of
        California Press.
Bateson, Gregory
    1958   Naven. Stanford: Stanford University Press.
Baur, John E.
    1959   The Health Seekers of Southern California, 1870–1900. San Marino,
        CA: The Huntington Library.
Bergson, Henri
    1913   Creative Evolution. New York: Henry Holt and Company.
Berkeley Holistic Health Center
    1978   Holistic Health Handbook. Berkeley: And/Or Press.
Bloomfield, Harold, and Robert Kory
    1978   The Holistic Way to Health and Happiness. New York: Simon and
        Schuster.

Blumer, Herbert
  1969   Social Movements. *In* Studies in Social Movements: A Social Psychological Perspective. Barry McLaughlin, ed. Pp. 8–29. New York: The Free Press.
Bohannan, Paul
  1963   Social Anthropology. New York: Holt, Rinehart and Winston.
Bonewits, P. E. Isaac
  1979   Real Magic: An Introductory Treatise on the Basic Principles of Yellow Magic. Berkeley: Creative Arts Book Company. 2nd edition.
Bowen, Eleanor Smith
  1964   Return to Laughter. Garden City: Anchor Press.
Bourguigon, Erika
  1973   A Framework for the Comparative Study of Altered States of Consciousness. *In* Religion. Altered States of Consciousness and Social Change. Erika Bourguigon, ed. Pp. 3–38. Columbus: Ohio State University Press.
Breen, Alan C.
  1979   Chiropractic. *In* A Visual Encyclopedia of Unconventional Medicine. Ann Hill, ed. Pp. 73–77. New York: Crown Publishers.
Bricklin, Mark
  1976   The Practical Encyclopedia of Natural Healing. Emmaus, PA: Rodale Press.
Bruce, F. F.
  1978   The Spreading Flame: The Rise and Progress of Christianity from the First Beginnings to the Conversion of the English. Greenwood, SC: The Attic Press.
Bürgel, J. Christoph
  1976   Secular and Religious Features of Medieval Arabic Medicine. *In* Asian Medical Systems. Charles Leslie, ed. Pp. 44–62. Berkeley: University of California Press.
Cantril, Hadley
  1963   The Psychology of Social Movements. New York: John Wiley and Sons.
Carrington, W.
  1972   The F. Mathias Alexander Technique: A Means of Understanding Man. Bulletin of Structural Integration 3(2): 44–62.
Carter, Mildred
  1980a   Hand Reflexology: A Key to Perfect Health. West Nyack, NY: Parker Publishing.
  1980b   Helping Yourself with Foot Reflexology. West Nyack, NY: Parker Publishing.

Chang, Stephan
    1978   Acupuncture: A Contemporary Look at an Ancient System. *In* Holistic Health Handbook. Berkeley Holistic Health Center, eds. Pp. 45–52. Berkeley: And/Or Press.
Chen, Graham
    1975   Neurohumors in Acupuncture. American Journal of Chinese Medicine 3(1): 27–43.
Chen, Gregory S.
    1977   Enkephalin, Drug Addiction and Acupuncture. American Journal of Chinese Medicine 5(1): 25–30.
Christopher, John R.
    1979   School of Natural Healing. Provo, UT: Biworld Publishers, Incorporated.
Chung, Shin-Ho, and Anthony Dickenson
    1980   Pain, Enkephalin and Acupuncture. Nature 283: 243–44.
Clopper, C. J. and E. S. Pearson
    1934   The Use of Confidence or Fiducial Limits Illustrated in the Case of the Binomial. Biometrika 26: 404–13.
Cobb, Ann Kuckelman
    1977   Pluralistic Legitimation of an Alternative Therapy System: The Case of Chiropractic. Medical Anthropology 1(4): 1–23.
Cohn, Norman
    1962   Medieval Millenarism: Its Bearing on the Comparative Study of Millenarian Movements. *In* Millenial Dreams in Action: Essays in Comparative Study. Comparative Studies in Society and History, Suppl. 2. Sylvia Thrupp, ed. pp. 31–43. The Hague: Mouton and Company.
    1970   The Pursuit of the Millennium. New York: Oxford University Press.
Concon, Archimedes
    1980   Introduction to the Principles of Homeopathy. American Journal of Acupuncture 8(1): 51–56.
Cotman, Carl, and James McGaugh
    1980   Behavioral Neuroscience. New York: Academic Press.
Coulter, Harris
    1973   Divided Legacy: A History of the Schism in Medical Thought. Volume III, Science and Ethics in American Medicine 1800–1914. Washington, D.C.: Wehawken Book Company.
    1975   Divided Legacy: A History of the Schism in Medical Thought. Volume I. The Patterns Emerge: Hippocrates to Paracelsus. Washington, D.C.: Wehawken Book Company.
    1977   Divided Legacy: A History of the Schism in Medical Thought. Volume II, Progress and Regress: J. B. van Helmont to Claude Bernard. Washington, D.C.: Wehawken Book Company.

1979   Homeopathic Medicine. *In* Ways of Health. David Sobel, ed. Pp. 289–310. New York: Harcourt, Brace, Jovanovich.

Cousins, Norman
1979   The Anatomy of an Illness as Perceived by the Patient. New York: W. W. Norton and Company.

Cowie, James and Julian Roebuck
1975   An Ethnography of a Chiropractic Clinic: Definitions of a Deviant Situation. New York: The Free Press.

Cox, Harvey
1978   Deep Structure in the Study of New Religions. *In* Understanding the New Religions. Jacob Needleman and George Bakers, eds. Pp. 122–30. New York: Seabury Press.

Crow, W. B.
1968   A History of Magic, Witchcraft and Occultism. London: The Aquarian Press.

Crozier, Ralph
1976   The Ideology of Medical Revivalism in Modern China. *In* Asian Medical Systems. Charles Leslie, ed. Pp. 341–55. Berkeley: University of California Press.

Das, Baba Hari and Dharma Sara Satsang
1978   Ayurveda: The Yoga of Health. *In* Holistic Health Handbook. Berkeley Holistic Health Center, eds. Pp. 53–61. Berkeley: And/Or Press.

Deliman, Tracy and John Smolowe, eds.
1982   Holistic Medicine. Reston, VA.: Reston Publishing Company.

Devereux, George
1980   Basic Problems of Ethnopsychiatry. Chicago: University of Chicago Press.

Diamond, Harvey
1979   The Totally Healthy Person: A Case against Medicine. Santa Monica: Golden Glow Publishers.

Diamond, Harvey and Marilyn
1985   Fit for Life. New York: Warner Books.

Diamond, Marilyn
1980   The Common Sense Guide to a New Way of Eating. Los Angeles: Golden Glow Publishers.

Dodds, E. R.
1951   The Greeks and the Irrational. Berkeley: University of California Press.
1965   Pagan and Christian in an Age of Anxiety: Some Aspects of Religious Experience from Marcus Aurelius to Constantine. Cambridge: University Press.

Dube, K. C.
  1978   Nosology and Therapy of Mental Illness. *In* Ayurveda. Comparative Medicine East and West 6: 209–28.
Duffy, John
  1979   The Healers: A History of American Medicine. Chicago: University of Illinois Press.
Dunn, Frederick L.
  1976   Traditional Medicine and Cosmopolitan Medicine as Adaptive Systems. *In* Asian Medical Systems. Charles Leslie, ed. Pp. 133–158. Berkeley: University of California Press.
Eliade, Mircea
  1964   Shamanism: Archaic Techniques of Ecstasy. New York: Bollingen Series; Pantheon Books.
  1976   Occultism, Witchcraft and Cultural Fashions: Essays in Comparative Religions. Chicago: University of Chicago Press.
Ellwood, Robert
  1973   Religions and Spiritual Groups in Modern America. Englewood Cliffs, NJ: Prentice-Hall.
  1978   Emergent Religion in America: A Historical Perspective. *In* Understanding the New Religions. Jacob Needleman and George Bakers, eds. Pp. 267–84. New York: Seabury Press.
  1979   Alternative Alters. Chicago: University of Chicago Press.
  1983   The American Theosophical Synthesis. *In* The Occult in America: New Historical Perspectives. Howard Kerr and Charles Crow, eds. Pp. 111–34. Chicago: University of Illinois Press.
Epstein, Perle
  1978   Kabbalah: The Way of the Jewish Mystic. New York: Samuel Weisner.
Evans-Pritchard, E. E.
  1964   Social Anthropology and Other Essays. New York: The Free Press of Glencoe.
Fadiman, James
  1981   Food and Nutrition. *In* Health for the Whole Person. Arthur Hastings, James Fadiman, and James Gordon, eds. Pp. 253–69. Toronto: Bantam Books.
Feldenkrais, Moshe
  1972   Awareness through Movement. New York: Harper and Row.
Ferguson, Marilyn
  1980   The Aquarian Conspiracy: Personal and Social Transformation in the 1980's. Los Angeles: J. P. Tarcher, Inc.
Filiozat, J.
  1964   The Classical Doctrine of Indian Medicine: Its Origins and its Greek Parallels. Nai Sarak, Delhi: Munshiram Mancharlal.

Foster, George, and Barbara Anderson
   1978   Medical Anthropology. New York: John Wiley and Sons.
Foucault, Michel
   1973   The Birth of the Clinic: An Archaeology of Medical Perception. New York: Pantheon Books.
Frager, Robert
   1981   Touch Working with the Body. *In* Health for the Whole Person. Arthur Hastings, James Fadiman, and James Gordon, eds. Pp. 215–32. Toronto: Bantam Books.
Freedland, Nat
   1972   The Occult Explosion. New York: G. P. Putnam's Sons.
Frend, W. H. C.
   1976   Religion Popular and Unpopular in the Early Christian Centuries. London: Variorum Press.
Galanti, Geri-Ann
   1981   The Psychic Reader as Shaman and Psychotherapist: The Interface between Clients' and Practitioners' Belief Systems in Los Angeles. Ph.D. Dissertation, Anthropology Department, Universityof California, Los Angeles.
Gall, John
   1975   Systemantics: How Systems Work and Especially How They Fail. New York: Quadrangle/ the New York Times Book Company.
Gandhi, Mahatma
   1978   The Health Guide. Trumansburg, NY: The Crossing Press.
Garfinkel, Harold
   1967   Studies in Ethnomethodology. Englewood Cliffs, NY: Prentice-Hall.
Garrison, Omar
   1973   Medical Astrology. New York: Warner Paberback Library.
Gerlach, Luther
   1980   Energy Wars and Social Change. *In* Predicting Sociocultural Change. Susan Abbott and John van Willigen, eds. pp. 76–94. Athens: University of Georgia Press.
Gerlach, Luther and Virginia Hine
   1973   Lifeway Leap: The Dynamics of Change in America. Minneapolis: University of Minnesota.
   1981   People, Power, Change: Movements of Social Transformation. Indianapolis: The Bobbs-Merrill Company.
Geyer, R. Felix
   1980   Alienation Theories: A General Systems Approach. Oxford: Pergamon Press.
Gilchrist, Keith
   1972   An Introduction to Structural Integration. Bulletin of Structural Integration 3(3): 4–10.

Goa, Hector
1982 The Healing Relationship. *In* Holistic Medicine. Tracy Deliman, and John Smolowe, eds. Pp. 245–48. Reston, VA.: Reston Publishing Company.
Goffman, Erving
1967 Interaction Ritual. Garden City, NY: Anchor Books, Doubleday and Company.
1970 Strategic Interaction. Philadelphia: University of Pennsylvania Press.
Goodman, Joseph
1979 Natural Hygiene. *In* A Visual Encyclopaedia of Unconventional Medicine. Ann Hill, ed. Pp. 138–39. New York: Crown Publishers.
Gordon, James S.
1981 The Paradigm of Holistic Medicine. *In* Health for the Whole Person. Arthur Hastings, James Fadiman and James Gordon, eds. pp. 3–40. Toronto: Bantam Books.
Green, Barry
1981 Body Therapies. *In* Handbook of Innovative Psychotherapies. Raymond Corsini, ed. Pp. 95–106. New York: Wiley-Interscience Publications.
Green, Jerry
1974 Medical Malpractice Laws as they Relate to Holistic Health Perspectives. Bulletin of Structural Integration 4(3): 16–20.
1978a Legal Issues in a Health Revolution. *In* Holistic Health Handbook. Berkeley Holistic Health Center, eds. Pp. 390–94. Berkeley: And/Or Press.
1978b Creating New Roles for Changing Times. *In* Wholistic Dimensions in Healing: A Resource Guide. Leslie Kaslof, ed. pp. 4–6. Garden City, NY: Doubleday and Company.
Gregory, Andre, and Wallace Shawn
1981 My Dinner with Andre. New York: Grove Press.
Grossinger, Richard
1980 Planet Medicine: From Stone Age Shamanism to Post-Industrial Healing. Garden City, NY: Anchor Press.
Gunji, Ryoichi
1973 Electric Acupuncture: Introduction to Simple Ryokoraku Treatment. Tokyo: Bunkodo Press.
Halprin, Anne, and Daria Halprin/Kalighi
1982 The Movement Dimension. *In* Holistic Medicine. Tracy Deliman and John Smolowe, eds. Pp. 70–92. Reston, VA.: Reston Publishing Company.
Harner, Michael
1980 The Way of the Shaman: A Guide to Power and Healing. San Francisco: Harper and Row.

Hastings, Arthur
  1981 Alternative Forms of Diagnosis. *In* Health for the Whole Person. Arthur Hastings, James Fadiman and James Gordon, eds. Pp. 460–83. Toronto: Bantam Books.
Henry, James
  1982 Possible Involvement of Endorphins in Altered States of Consciousness. Ethos 10(4): 394–408.
Hill, Lawrence
  1930 Santa Barbara, Tierra Adorada: A Community History. Los Angeles: Security First National Bank of Los Angeles.
Hine, Robert
  1983 California's Utopian Colonies. Berkeley: University of California Press.
Hine, Virginia
  1977 The Basic Paradigm of a Future Socio-Cultural System. World Issues 11(2): 19–22.
  1980 How do we get from Here to There? Paper presented to the Hutchins Center for the Study of Democratic Institutions in association with the University of California, Santa Barbara. May 29, 1980.
Hoffman, Edward, and W. Edward Mann
  1980 The Man Who Dreamed of Tomorrow: A Conceptual Biography of Wilhelm Reich. Los Angeles: J. P. Tarcher Press.
Huard, Pierre, and Ming Wong
  1968 Chinese Medicine. New York: World University Library.
Huxley, Aldous
  1969 Ends and Means. London: Chatto and Windus Ltd.
Jackson, J. A.
  1970 Professions and Professionalization. *In* Professions and Professionalization, J. A. Jackson, ed. Cambridge: Cambridge University Press.
Jensen, Bernard
  1952 The Science and Practice of Iridology. Provo, UT: Biworld Publications
Jilek, Wolfgang
  1982 Altered States of Consciousness in North American Indian Ceremonials. Ethos 10(4): 326–42.
Jones, Mario
  1978 Astrology of Medicine. *In* Wholistic Dimensions in Healing: A Resource Guide. Leslie Kaslof, ed. Pp. 162–64. Garden City, NY: Doubleday and Company.
Kalson, Carol, and Stan Kalson
  1979 Holistic H.E.L.P. Handbook. Phoenix, AZ: International Holistic Center, Inc.

Kao, Frederick
1973 Acupuncture Therapeutics. New Haven, CT.: Eastern Press.
Kaslof, Leslie, ed.
1978 Wholistic Dimensions in Healing: A Resource Guide. Garden City, NY: Doubleday and Company.
Kaufman, Martin
1971 Homeopathy in America: The Rise and Fall of a Medical Heresy. Baltimore: Johns Hopkins Press.
Kaufmann, Draper
1980 Systems One: An Introduction to Systems Thinking. Minneapolis: Future Systems, Inc.
Kellogg, John Harvey
1929 The Art of Massage. Battle Creek, MI.: Modern Medicine Publishing.
Kelley, Charles and Julie Wright
n.d. Radix Neo-Reichian Education. Unpublished Brochure.
Kloss, Jethro
1971 Back to Eden: A Human Interest Story of Health and Restoration to be Found in Herb, Root and Bark. New York: Lancer books.
Koster, Donald Nelson
1975 Transcendentalism in America. Boston: Twayne Publishers.
Kriege, Theodor
1980 Fundamental Basis of Irisdiagnosis. A. W. Priest, transl. Romford, Essex: LN Fowler and Company.
Kunz, Barbara, and Kevin Kunz
1982 A Complete Guide to Reflexology. Englewood Cliffs, NJ: Prentice-Hall, Inc.
Langfield, A. W.
1979 Exploring Socialization through the Interpersonal Transaction Group. *In* Constructs of Sociality and Individuality. P. Stringer and D. Bannister, eds. New York: Academic Press.
Lathim, Kim and Rod Lathim
1975 The Spirit of the Big Yellow House. Santa Barbara: located Santa Barbara County Library.
Leblanc, Steven
1973 Two Points of Logic Concerning Data, Hypotheses, General Law and Systems. *In* Research and Theory in Current Archaeology. Charles Redman, ed. Pp. 199–214. New York: John Wiley and Sons.
Leslie, Charles
1975 Pluralism and Integration in the Indian and Chinese Medical systems. *In* Medicine in Chinese Cultures. Arthur Kleinman, ed. Pp. 401–18.
1976a Asian Medical Systems: A Comparative Study. Berkeley: University of California Press.

1976b   The Ambiguities of Medical Revivalism in Modern India. *In* Asian Medical Systems. Charles Leslie, ed. Pp. 356–67. Berkeley: University of California Press.

Levine, Edwin Burton
1971   Hippocrates. New York: Twayne Publishers.

Levine, Jon. D., Newton Gorgon, and Howard Fields
1978   The Mechanism of Placebo Analgesia. The Lancet 2: 654–57.

Lewis, Roy and Angus Maude
1952   Professional People. London: Phoenix House, Ltd.

Lloyd, G. E. R.
1978   Hippocratic Writings. New York: Penguin Books.

Mahdihassan, S.
1979   Indian and Chinese Cosmic Elements. American Journal of Chinese Medicine. 7(4): 316–23.

Malinowki Bronislaw
1967   A Diary in the Strict Sense of the World. New York: Harcourt, Brace and World, Inc.
1978   Coral Gardens and Their Magic: A Study of the Methods of Tilling the Soil and of Agricultural Rites in the Trobriand Islands (Two volumes bound as one). New York: Dover Publications, Inc.

Mandler, George
1984   Mind and Body: The Psychology of Emotions and Stress. New York: W Norton and Company.

Marchetti, Veeda
1985   Marching Back to Jerusalem: Ecstatic Religion in Middle Class America. Ph.D. dissertation, Department of Anthropology, University of California, Santa Barbara.

Mattson, Phyllis
1977   Holistic Health: an Overview. Phoenix: New Directions in the Study of Man 1(2): 36–43.
1982   Holistic Health in Perspective. Palo Alto, CA: Mayfield Publishing Company.

Maykovich, Minado K.
1980   Medical Sociology. Sherman Oaks, CA: Alfred Publishing Company.

McGarey, William A.
1978   Edgar Cayce and Wholistic Medicine. *In* Wholistic Dimensions in Healing: A Resource Guide. Leslie Kaslof, ed. Pp. 197–99. Garden City: Doubleday.

Mead, G. R. S.
1967   The Doctrine of the Subtle Body in Western Thought (first published 1919). Madras, India: Theosophical Publishing House.

Mead, Margaret
    1964   Continuities in Cultural Evolution. Clinton, MA.: The Colonial
    Press, Inc.
    1977   Letters from the Field: 1925–1975. New York: Harper and Row.
Meeks, Wayne
    1983   The First Urban Christians: The Social World of the Apostle Paul.
    New Haven, CT.: Yale University Press.
Molgaard, Craig Allen
    1979   New Age Hunters and Gatherers, Ph.D. dissertation, Anthropology
    Department, University of California, Berkeley.
Montgomery, Edward
    1976   Systems and Medical Practitioners of a Tamil Town. *In* Asian Medi-
    cal Systems. Charles Leslie, ed. Pp. 272–84. Berkeley: University of Cali-
    fornia Press.
Montagna, F. Joseph
    1979   Peoples Desk Reference. Volumes I and II. Traditional Herbal For-
    mulas. Lake Oswego, OR: Quest for Truth Publications, Inc.
Murphy, Jane
    1964   Psychotherapeutic Aspects of Shamanism on St. Lawrence Island. *In*
    Magic, Faith and Healing. Ari Kiev, ed. New York: The Free Press.
Needham, Joseph
    1970   Clerks and Craftsmen in China and the West. London: Cambridge
    University Press.
Needham, Joseph, and Lu Gwei-Djen
    1969   Chinese Medicine. *In* Medicine and Culture. F. N. L. Poynter, ed.
    Pp. 255–314. London: Wellcome Institute of the History of Medicine.
    1980   Celestial Lancets: A History and Rationale of Acupuncture and
    Moxa. Cambridge: Cambridge University Press.
Numbers, Ronald
    1977   Do it Yourself the Sectarian Way. *In* Medicine without Doctors.
    Guenter Risse, Ronald Numbers and Judith Leavitt, eds. Pp. 49–72. New
    York: Science History Publication.
Obeyeskere, Gananath
    1976   The Impact of Ayurvedic Ideas on the Culture and the Individual in
    Sri Lanka. *In* Asian Medical Systems. Charles Leslie, ed. Pp. 201–26.
    Berkeley: University of California Press.
    1977   The Theory and Practice of Psychological Medicine in the Ayurvedic
    Tradition. Culture, Medicine and Psychiatry 1(2): 155–82.
Odum, Eugene
    1966   Ecology. New York: Holt, Rinehart and Winston.
Orne, Martin
    1980   Hypnotic Control of Pain: Toward a Clarification of the Different

Psychological Processes Involved. *In* Pain. John Bonica, ed. Pp. 154–72. New York: Raven Press.

Otsuka, Yasuo

1976   Chinese Traditional Medicine in Japan. *In* Asian Medical Systems. Charles Leslie, ed. Pp. 322–40. Berkeley: University of California Press.

Pagels, Elaine

1980   Gnostic Texts Revive Ancient Contraversies. The Center Magazine 13(5): 53–64.

1981   The Gnostic Gospels. New York: Vintage Books.

Palumbo, Dennis

1977   Statistics in Political and Behavioral Science (Revised Edition). New York: Columbia University Press.

Pannetier, Pierre

1978   Polarity Therapy. *In* Wholistic Dimensions in Healing: A Resource Guide. Leslie Kaslof, ed. Pp. 216–18. Garden City, New York: Doubleday and Company.

Pavalko, Ronald

1971   Sociology of Occupations and Professions. Itasca, IL.: F. E. Peacock Publishers, Inc.

Pelletier, Kenneth

1977   Mind as Healer, Mind as Slayer. New York: Dell Publishing Company.

Peng, Lee, M. M. P. Yang, S. H. Kok, and Y. K. Woo

1978   Endorphin Release: A Possible Mechanism of Acupuncture Analgesia. Comparative Medicine East and West 6(1): 57–60.

Perls, Frederick S.

1969   Gestalt Therapy Verbatim. Lafayette, CA: Real People Press.

Pessar, Patricia

1980   Revolution, Salvation, Extermination: The Future of Millenarianism in Brazil. *In* Predicting Sociocultural Change. Susan Abbott and John van Willigen, eds. pp. 95–114. Athens: University of Georgia Press.

Peters, Larry and Douglass Price-Williams

1980   Towards an Experiential Analysis of Shamanism. American Ethnologist 7(3): 397–418.

Platt, John

1969   Lock-ins and Multiple Lock-ins in Collective Behavior. American Scientist 57(2): 96–100A.

1970   Hierarchical Restructuring. General Systems 15: 49–54.

1971   Notes Toward a Theory of Behavioral Modification and Social Change.Unpublished Draft. Files of the Author.

1973   Social Traps. American Psychologist 28(8): 641–51.

1975   The Future of Social Crises. The Futurist 9(5): 266–68.

1980   Nature, Nurture, Networks: Three Social Organizing Principles. Paper presented at AAAS-SGSR Symposium on Living Sciences. San Francisco. January 8, 1980.

Pomeranz, Bruce
1982   Acupuncture and the Endorphins. Ethos 10(4): 385–93.

Porkert, Manfred
1976   The Intellectual and Social Impulses behind the Evolution of Traditional Chinese Medicine. *In* Asian Medical Systems. Charles Leslie, ed. Pp. 63–81. Berkeley: University of California Press.
1980   The Theoretical Foundations of Chinese Medicine: Systems of Correspondance. Cambridge: Massachusetts Institute of Technology Press.

Powdermaker, Hortense
1967   Stranger and Friend: The Way of an Anthropologist. New York: Norton Publishing.

Prakash, Buddha
1964   India and the World. Hoshiarpur: Vishveshvaranand Vedic Research Institute.

Prince, Raymond
1982   Shamans and Endorphins. Ethos 10(4): 409–23.

Revolutionary Health Committee of Hunan Province
1977   A Barefoot Doctor's Manual. Seattle: Madrona Publishers.

Reich, Wilhelm
1973   Ether, God, and Devil: Cosmic Superimposition. New York: Farrar, Straus and Giroux.
1978   The Function of the Orgasm: Sex Economic Problems of Biological Energy. New York: Pocket Books.

Rindos, David
1984   The Origins of Agriculture: An Evolutionary Perspective. New York: Academic Press.

Rogers, Spencer
1982   The Shaman: His Symbols and His Healing Power. Springfield, IL.: Charles C. Thomas.

Roth, Julius
1976   Health Purifiers and Their Enemies: A Study of the Natural Health Movement in the United States with a Comparison to its Counterpart in Germany. New York: Prodist.

Salmon, Merrilee
1982   Philosophy and Archaeology. New York: Academic Press.

Salmon, Marrilee, and Wesley Salmon
1979   Alternative Models of Scientific Explanation. American Anthropologist 81: 61–74.

Samuels, Mike, and Nancy Samuels
1980 Seeing with the Mind's Eye: The History, Techniques and Uses of Visualization. New York: Random House.

Sanyal, P. K.
1964 A Story of Medicine and Pharmacy in India. Calcutta: Navana Printing Works Private Limited.

Saunders, J. B. de C.
1963 The Transition from Ancient Egyptian to Greek Medicine: Lawrence: University of Kansas Press.

Schulz, Will
1981 Holistic Education. *In* Handbook of Innovative Psychotherapies. Raymond Corsini, ed. Pp. 378–88. New York: Wiley-Interscience Publications.

Selinsky, Phillip
n.d. Workbook of Acupuncture Point Location. Unpublished Manuscript. Author's Files.
1982 Newsletter for the Institute of Holistic Studies. August 1982.
1984 Newsletter for the Institute of Holistic Studies. August 1984.

Senf, Bernd
1979 Wilhelm Reich, Discoverer of Acupuncture Energy. American Journal of Acupuncture 2(7): 109–18.

Shames, Richard, and Chuck Sterin
1978 Healing with Mind Power. Emmaus, PA: Rodale Press.

Sharma, C. H.
1979 Ayurvedic Medicine. *In* A Visual Encyclopeadia of Unconventional Medicine. Ann Hill, ed. Pp. 17–21. New York: Crown Publishers.

Shorr, Joseph
1981 Psycho-Imagination Therapy. *In* Handbook of Innovative Psychotherapies. Raymond Corsini, ed. Pp. 694–708. New York: Wiley-Interscience Publications.

Silverberg, Robert
1976 Shadrach in the Furnace. Indianapolis: The Bobbs-Merrill Company.

Skinner, B. F.
1981 Selection by Consequences. Science 213: 501–4.

Skultans, Vieda
1976 Empathy and Healing: Aspects to Spiritualist Healing. *In* Social Anthropology and Medicine. J. B. Loudon, ed. Pp. 190–222. New York: Academic Press.

Snyder, Paul
1980 Health and Human Nature. Radnor, PA: Chilton Book Company.

Stanford Research Institute
1960 Chiropractic in California. Los Angeles: The Haynes Foundation.

Stark, Eli, and McFarlane Tilley
  1975   Osteopathic Medicine. Acton, MA: Publishing Sciences.
Stein, Larry, and James Belluzzi
  1979   Brain Endorphins: Possible Mediators of Pleasurable States. *In* Endorphins in Mental Health Research. Earl Usdin, William Bunney, and Nathan Kline, eds. Pp. 375–89. New York: Oxford University Press.
Steiner, Rudolf
  1973   The Occult Movement in the Nineteenth Century and its Relation to Modern culture. D. S. Osmond, transl. London: Rudolf Steiner Press.
Stone, Randolph
  1953   A course in Manipulative Therapy with Principles and Illustrations of the New Energy Concepts of the Healing Art. Olga, WA: Polarity Institute Alive Fellowship.
  1957   Energy: The Vital Polarity in the Healing Art. Olga, WA: Polarity Institute Alive Fellowship.
  1978   Health Building: The Conscious Art of Living Well. Olga, WA: Polarity Institute Alive Fellowship.
Talmon, Yonina
  1965   Pursuit of the Millennium: The Relation between Religion and Social Change. *In* Reader in Comparative Religion: An Anthropological Approach. 2nd ed. William Lessa and Evon Vogt, eds. pp. 522–36. New York: Harper and Row.
Tappan, Frances M.
  1978   Healing Massage Techniques: A Study of Eastern and Western Methods. Reston, VA.: Reston Publishing Company.
Taylor, Pat Ellis
  1981   Border Healing Woman: The Story of Jewel Babb. Austin: University of Texas Press.
Teeguarden, Iona
  1978   Acupressure Way of Health: Jin Shin Do. Tokyo: Japan Publication.
Teeguarden, Iona and Ron Teeguarden
  1978a   Jin Shin Do: Acupressure Workbook. Basic Course. Santa Monica: The Acupressure Workshop.
  1978b   Jin Shin Do: Acupressure Workbook. Intermediate Course. Santa Monica: The Acupressure Workshop.
  1978c   Jin Shin Do: Acupressure Workbook. Advanced Course. Santa Monica: The Acupressure Workshop.
Teeguarden, Ron
  1980a   The Five Elemental Energies: The Taoist Theory of the Cycles of Nature and Its Practical Utilization in the Various Chinese Healthways. Santa Monica: The Acupressure Workshop.
  1980b   Chinese Tonic Herbs. Santa Monica: The Acupressure Workshop.

Textor, Robert
    1980   A Handbook on Ethnographic Futures Research. Third edition, Version A. Stanford, CA: Cultural and Educational Futures Research Project. Schoold of Education and Department of Anthropology.
Tharp, Roland, and David Watson
    1977   Self-Directed Behavior: Self-modification for Personal Adjustment. Monterey: Brooks/Cole Publishing.
Thie, John
    1979   Touch for Health. Marina del Rey, CA: DeVorss
Thomas, Lewis
    1981   Medicine without Science. The Atlantic Monthly. 247(4): 40–42.
Thorwald, Jürgen
    1962   Science and Secrets of Early Medicine. London: Thames and Hudson.
Thrupp, Sylvia
    1962   Millennial Dreams in Action. *In* Millennial Dreams in Action: Essays in Comparative Studies. Comparative Studies in Society and History, Suppl. 2. Sylvia Thrupp, ed. pp. 11–30. The Hague: Mouton and Company.
Toguchi, Masaru
    1974   Complete Guide to Acupuncture. New York: Frederick Fell, Publishers.
Tompkins, Walter
    1975   Santa Barbara: Past and Present. Santa Barbara: Tecolote Books.
Treacher, Andrew, and Peter Wright
    1982   The Problem of Medical Knowledge: Examination of the Social Construction of Medicine. Edinburgh: Edinburgh University Press.
Turner, C. and M. N. Hodge
    1970   Occupations and Professions. *In* Professions and Professionalization, J. A. Jackson, ed. Pp. 17–50. Cambridge: Cambridge University Press.
United States Department of Commerce. Bureau of the Census
    1980   Census of Population and Housing, Washington: United States Government Printing Office.
Unschuld, Paul Ulrich
    1973   Die Praxis des Traditionellen Chinesischen Heilsystems. Weisbaden: Franz Steiner Verlag.
    1976   The Social Organization and Ecology of Medical Practice in Taiwan. *In* Asian Medical Systems. Charles Leslie, ed. Pp. 300–21. Berkeley: University of California Press.
    1977a   The Development of Medical Pharmeceutical Thought in China. Part I. Comparative Medicine East and West 5(2): 109–15.
    1977b   The Development of Medical Pharmeceutical Thought in China. Part II. Comparative Medicine East and West 5(3): 211–31.

1979   Medical Ethics in Imperial China. Berkeley: University of California Press.

Upadhyahya, B. S.
1973   Feeders of Indian Culture. New Delhi: People's Publishing House.

Vieth, Ilza
1972   Huang Ti Nei Ching Su Wen (The Yellow Emperor's Classic of Internal Medicine). Berkeley: University of California Press.

Vithoulkas, George
1980   The Science of Homeopathy. New York: Grove Press.
1981   Homeopathy: Medicine of the New Man. New York: Arco Publishing.

Walker, Benjamin
1983   Gnosticism. Wellingborough, Northhamptonshire: The Aquarian Press.

Walker, Helen, and Joseph Lev
1953   Statistical Inference. New York: Holt, Rinehart and Winston.

Wallace, A. F. C.
1956   Revitalization Movements. American Anthropologist 58: 264–81.

Wang, Xue-Tai
1979   The Origin and Development of Chinese Acupuncture and Moxabustion. American Journal of Acupuncture. 7(4): 293–304.

Wax, Rosalie
1971   Doing Fieldwork. Warnings and Advice. Chicago: University of Chicago Press.

Weber, Max
1968   On Charismatic Institution Building. Selected Papers. S. N. Eisenstadt, ed. Chicago: University of Chicago Press.

Weeks, Nora
1979   Bach Flower Remedies. *In* A Visual Encyclopeadia of Unconventional Medicine. Ann Hill, ed. Pp. 122–23. New York: Crown Publishers.

Wei, Ling Y.
1979   Scientific Advance in Acupuncture. American Journal of Chinese Medicine 7(1): 53–75.

Weir, Sir John
1972   Homeopathy: An Explanation of its Principles. Bulletin of Structural Integration 3(3): 28–54.

Whiteside, Robert
n.d.   Personology. Unpublished Manual. Interstate College of Personology.

Wilk, Chester
1976   Chiropractic Speaks Out: A Reply to Medical Propaganda, Bigotry and Ignorance. Park Ridge, IL: Wilk Publishing Company.

Wilson, Robert Anton
1978   Cosmic Trigger: The Final Secret of the Illuminati. New York: Pocket Books.

1981   Masks of the Illuminati. New York: Timescape/Pocket Books.
Yamamoto, Schizuko
1979   Barefoot Shiatsu. Tokyo: Japan Publications.
Yang, Mabel, and S. H. Kok
1979   Further Study of the Neurohumoral Factor, Endorphin, in the Mechanism of Acupuncture Analgesia. American Journal of Chinese medicine 7(2): 143–48.
Young, James Henry
1977   Patent Medicines and the Self-Help Syndrome. *In* Medicine Without Doctors. Guenter Risse, Ronald Numbers and Judith Leavitt, eds. Pp. 95–116. New York: Science History Press.
Zabarenko, Ralph, and Lucy Zabarenko
1978   The Doctor Tree: Developmental Stages in the Growth of Physicians. Pittsburgh: University of Pittsburgh Press.
Zeeman, E. C.
1977   Catastrophe Theory: Selected Papers 1972–1977. London: Addison-Wesley Publishing Company.
1982   Decision Making and Evolution. *In* Theory and Explanation in Archaeology. Colin Renfrew, M. Rowlands, and Barbara Segraves, eds. Pp. 315–46. New York: Academic Press.